Value Driven Healthcare
and Geriatric Medicine

AF148094

James S. Powers

Value Driven Healthcare and Geriatric Medicine

Implications for Today's Changing
Health System

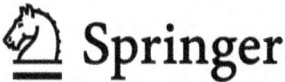 Springer

James S. Powers, MD
Vanderbilt University School of Medicine
Tennessee Valley Healthcare System
Geriatric Research Education and Clinical Center
Nashville, TN
USA

ISBN 978-3-319-77056-7   ISBN 978-3-319-77057-4   (eBook)
https://doi.org/10.1007/978-3-319-77057-4

Library of Congress Control Number: 2018939438

© Springer International Publishing AG, part of Springer Nature 2018
This work is subject to copyright. All rights are reserved by the Publisher, whether the whole or part of the material is concerned, specifically the rights of translation, reprinting, reuse of illustrations, recitation, broadcasting, reproduction on microfilms or in any other physical way, and transmission or information storage and retrieval, electronic adaptation, computer software, or by similar or dissimilar methodology now known or hereafter developed.
The use of general descriptive names, registered names, trademarks, service marks, etc. in this publication does not imply, even in the absence of a specific statement, that such names are exempt from the relevant protective laws and regulations and therefore free for general use.
The publisher, the authors and the editors are safe to assume that the advice and information in this book are believed to be true and accurate at the date of publication. Neither the publisher nor the authors or the editors give a warranty, express or implied, with respect to the material contained herein or for any errors or omissions that may have been made. The publisher remains neutral with regard to jurisdictional claims in published maps and institutional affiliations.

Printed on acid-free paper

This Springer imprint is published by the registered company Springer International Publishing AG part of Springer Nature.
The registered company address is: Gewerbestrasse 11, 6330 Cham, Switzerland

Preface

The US healthcare system is undergoing a value-based transformation. Value-driven healthcare has three goals: to improve access to healthcare by increasing healthcare insurance coverage, to improve the patient's experience and quality of care, and to slow the rate of increase in healthcare costs. The main premise of this book is that value-based purchasing for healthcare is likely to remain a constant feature of the healthcare horizon. The second is that value-based purchasing drives quality metrics which are publicly reported and serve as important levers for changes in healthcare delivery.

Value-based purchasing is a demand side strategy to reward quality in healthcare delivery. Value-based purchasing involves cost considerations and includes the actions of employers, the public sector, health plans, and individual consumers in making healthcare decisions. Effective healthcare services and high performing healthcare providers are incentivized to provide quality outcomes and to control cost.

The opportunities and challenges involved in value-based transformation are real and substantial. The US has the world's largest observable discrepancy between the amount spent in healthcare and the health status of the population, but it is also positioned with the knowledge needed for improving value and outcomes. Accelerating the movement toward a reward system based on results is possible. The urgency is as compelling as the opportunities. There is no easy fix or simple budgetary adjustment that will resolve excessive healthcare spending or cost inefficiencies in multiple components of the health system. The complexity and magnitude of the issues as well as the promise for gain call for vigorous leadership.

Geriatric patients consume a disproportionate share of healthcare resources. CMS directs Medicare and drives geriatric healthcare models. All other insurers generally model CMS/Medicare guidelines. Innovative geriatric care models which demonstrate improved outcomes and cost moderation can be scaled and lessons learned used to create new healthcare models.

This book traces the origins of value-based purchasing and current geriatric care models. It also discusses healthcare accountability and risk sharing. The audience includes geriatric healthcare professionals as well as a wider audience interested in healthcare models and value driven healthcare from a policy, economic, and ethical perspective.

Nashville, TN, USA   James S. Powers

Acknowledgment

Laura M. Keohane, Ph.D., M.S., is an assistant professor in the Department of Health Policy at Vanderbilt University School of Medicine. She investigates health policy issues related to aging and disability with a focus on dual-eligible beneficiaries, post-acute care services, and long-term services and supports. She holds a Ph.D. in health services research from Brown University and a M.S. in health policy and management from the Harvard School of Public Health. Her involvement was invaluable in finding data sources and describing low income, special-needs elderly populations.

Contents

About the Author

James S. Powers, M.D. is Professor of Medicine at Vanderbilt University School of Medicine and Associate Clinical Director at the Tennessee Valley Healthcare System, Geriatrics Research Education and Clinical Center (TVHS GRECC), Nashville, TN. He is the Geriatrics Fellowship Program Director. The views expressed are based on his experience of over three decades consulting, developing, evaluating, and sustaining primary care and geriatric healthcare models and educational programs throughout the Mid-South. Dr. Powers focuses on quality improvement and evaluating educational and clinical outcomes, maintains a large practice, and teaches geriatrics to healthcare professionals of all disciplines. He writes from the perspective of a physician speaking to colleagues, administrators, policy makers, and educators on the value of the geriatrics perspective in healthcare planning and delivery.

Chapter 1
Value-Based Healthcare Transformation

Abstract The United States spends more on healthcare than any other developed nation, yet it ranks 37th in total health outcomes. Healthcare inflation risks solvency of the Medicare Trust Fund and spending approaches 20% of the gross domestic product (GDP). Historic policy trends to control healthcare costs are detailed. The aims of value-based healthcare transformation are to (1) improve access, (2) improve quality, and (3) slow the rate of healthcare cost increase. Healthcare inflation has slowed with the advent of value-based healthcare purchasing.

The United States spends more on healthcare than any other developed country (Fig. 1.1). Since the 1960s, healthcare growth exceeded GDP, increasing from 5% of GDP in 1960 to 16.4% of GDP in 2013 [1]. After adjusting for inflation and using the GDP price index, average health spending growth was 5.5% between 1960 and 2013 compared to a 3.1% growth in the GDP [2].

Healthcare costs have risen at an unsustainable rate exceeding both education and defense spending. The United States falls at 37 in overall health outcomes, trailing many nations in infant mortality, life expectancy, patient safety, healthcare access, disease management, and measures of health disparities [2]. Yet there are serious mismatches between cost outcomes and distribution of health resources

© Springer International Publishing AG, part of
Springer Nature 2018
J. S. Powers, *Value Driven Healthcare and Geriatric Medicine*,
https://doi.org/10.1007/978-3-319-77057-4_1

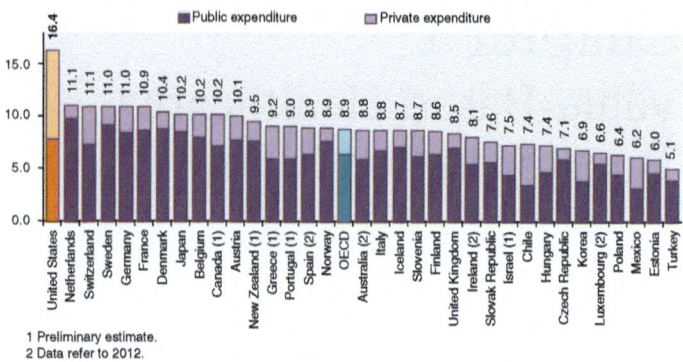

1 Preliminary estimate.
2 Data refer to 2012.

FIGURE 1.1 Total health expenditures as a share of GDP (2013)

in the United States. This combination of high cost, poor outcomes, and geographic variation in the Medicare fee-for-service population has fueled the perception of an inefficient US healthcare system which lacks transparency (Fig. 1.2). The reality of maldistribution of resources, cost, quality, and outcomes is driving value-based care transformation. By this we mean process standardization, more organized and coordinated systems focusing on cost consciousness and medical decisions, as well as greater price and quality transparency.

There are other reasons for healthcare transformation and a paradigm shift in healthcare delivery. The Medicare Hospital Insurance Trust Fund faces insolvency. Depending on healthcare inflation, there is a predicted 2028 intermediate estimate for Health Insurance Trust Fund depletion (Fig. 1.3). Under low cost assumptions, trust fund assets could continue to increase throughout the entire projection through 2035, but under a high cost assumption the fund depletion could occur as early as 2022 [3]. The Congressional Budget Office (CBO) reports that healthcare spending is projected to continue to grow [4] (Fig. 1.4) at an average rate of 5.6% per year (2016 to 2025) [5]. It was inevitable that serious consideration to slowing the rate of healthcare inflation and improving the quality of care would dominate the healthcare landscape. The urgency is compelling and the opportunities for improvement are legion.

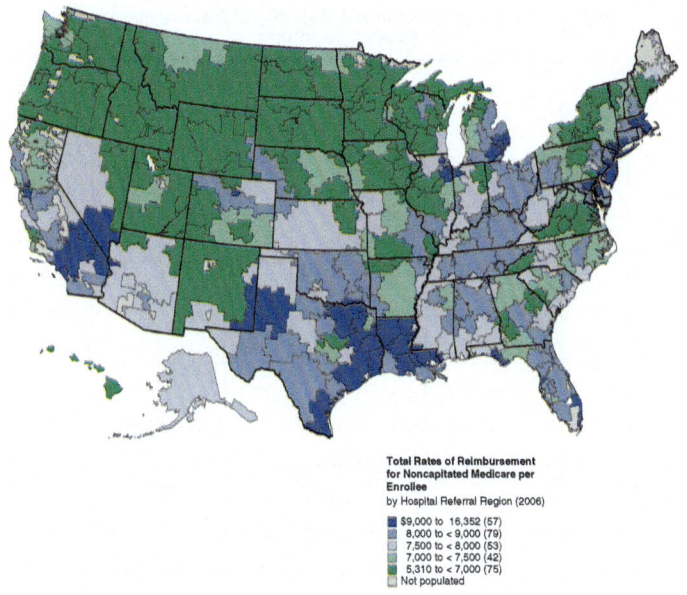

Total Rates of Reimbursement
for Noncapitated Medicare per
Enrollee
by Hospital Referral Region (2006)

■ $9,000 to 16,352 (57)
  8,000 to < 9,000 (79)
  7,500 to < 8,000 (53)
  7,000 to < 7,500 (42)
■ 5,310 to < 7,000 (75)
  Not populated

FIGURE 1.2 National variation in Medicare spending (Fisher ES, Goodman DC, Skinner JS, Bronner KK. Health care spending, quality and outcomes. Hanover, NH: Trustees of Dartmouth College, February 27, 2009. http://www.dartmouthatlas.org/downloads/reports/Spending_Brief_022709.pdf)

The United States is undergoing a value-driven healthcare transformation with three goals: (1) to improve access to health care by increasing healthcare insurance coverage, (2) to improve the patient's experience and quality of care, and (3) to slow the rate of increase in healthcare costs. Defining the provisions of healthcare coverage, its financing, and regulation remains a heated debate [6] although most Americans view many elements of healthcare transformation positively [7]. In contrast, there is strong agreement on all fronts that policy action is needed to address rising medical costs, and to assure the provision of quality medical care. Regardless of structural modifications of government financing of health care, value-based purchasing for health care is likely to remain a constant feature of the healthcare horizon.

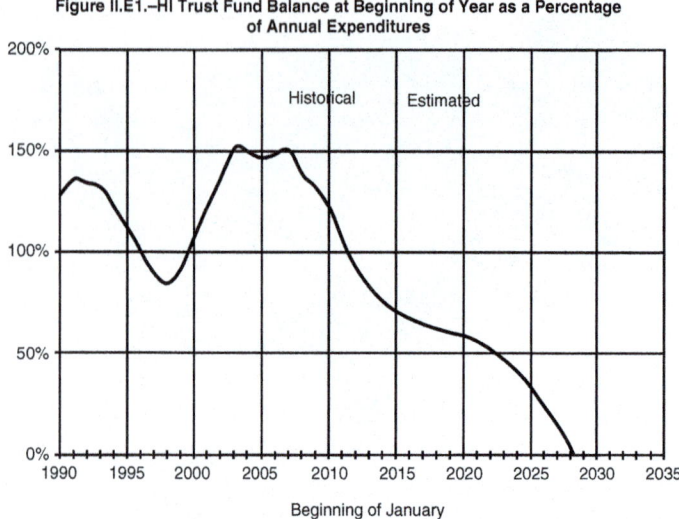

FIGURE 1.3 Health Insurance Trust Fund Balance [2] from the 2016 Trustees Report [4]

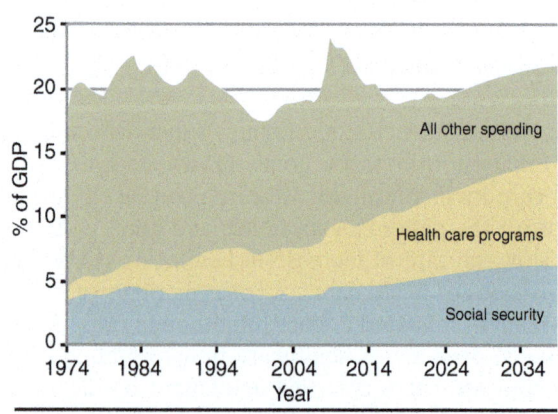

All other spending includes other mandatory spending and discretionary spending (including defense and nondefense). Data are from the Congressional Budget Office. GDP indicated gross domestic product.

FIGURE 1.4 Historical and projected federal healthcare spending [4]

A closer inspection of US healthcare costs is instructive. Per capita national health expenditures were $10,384 and total national health expenditures were $3.3 trillion in 2016, with total national health expenditures as a percent of GDP 17.9% [5]. Medicare comprised 20% of total healthcare expenditures and 44% of government healthcare expenditures, while Medicaid comprised 37% of government healthcare expenditures [8]. The percent of national health expenditures for hospital care was 32.3% and the percent of national health expenditures for nursing care facilities and continuing care retirement communities was 4.9%. National health expenditures for physician and clinical services were 19.8% and the percent of national health expenditures for prescription drugs was 10.1% (2015) [9].

However, aggregated measures of healthcare spending do not adequately represent the effect of rising costs on families. A healthcare affordability index has been proposed which relates health insurance costs to household incomes over time [10]. This index, excluding out-of-pocket expenses, is comprised of total healthcare premiums (employer and household) associated with mean employer sponsored health insurance divided by the median income of US households. It shows an increase from 14.2% of median income in 1999 to 30.7% of median income in 2016 [3, 11]. Direct consumer contributions to premiums rose from 9.2% in 1999 to 18.4% in 2016, making healthcare insurance premiums more costly than food expenditures for the average consumer [12]. Indeed in 2007, 62% of bankruptcies were due to medical bills [13]. The rapid growth of healthcare expenses relative to growth in the economy has translated into an increasing financial burden for households, employers, as well as state and federal government.

Geriatric patients consume a disproportionate share of healthcare resources. CMS directs Medicare and drives geriatric healthcare models. All other insurers generally model CMS/Medicare guidelines for geriatric consumers. Innovative geriatric care models which demonstrate improved outcomes and cost moderation can be scaled and lessons learned used to create new healthcare models. Major changes in healthcare financing and delivery are inevitable with emphasis on reducing unnecessary expenses and costs associated with little or no outcome benefit. The most important challenge for healthcare policy for the foreseeable future is to bring more cost discipline to bear on the provision of medical services, which will help to ensure that what is spent truly improves the health of patients.

Value-based purchasing is a demand-side strategy to reward quality in healthcare delivery. Value-based purchasing involves cost considerations and includes the actions of employers, the public sector, health plans, and individual consumers in making healthcare decisions. Effective healthcare services and high-performing healthcare providers are incentivized to provide quality outcomes and to control cost. Value-based purchasing has the potential to drive quality metrics serving as important levers for changes in healthcare delivery [14].

What is the evidence that value-based purchasing has been effective in addressing the three aims of healthcare transformation: (1) improved access to enhanced quality of care, (2) improved patient's experience and quality of care, and (3) slowing of the rate of healthcare cost growth?

With Respect to Access

Improved access has occurred from 2000 to 2016. According to CMS some 20 million previously uninsured individuals under age 65 now have health insurance as a result of the Affordable Care Act of 2010. This represents an approximate 50% reduction in the uninsured population so now less than 9% of Americans lack health insurance [15]. Improved access is important as lack of healthcare insurance is associated with delayed care and worse healthcare outcomes. High-risk and special-needs patients as well as indigent populations remain highly vulnerable to access barriers.

With Regard to Quality of Care

Since 2010, there have been a number of positive changes in the quality of health care in the United States. There has been a 10% reduction in the 30-day hospital readmission rate among US hospitals. Health status quality metrics for accountable care organizations (ACOs) have showed a growth in overall improvement in meeting objectives from 70 to 84%. Many new healthcare models have been stimulated and disseminated including ACOs, patient-centered medical homes, bundled disease state payments, and other provider-shared risk programs [16].

Transparent quality reporting is associated with improved outcomes as well. Nursing Home Compare has driven reduction in restraint utilization and antipsychotic prevalence (Chap. 3). These initial successes have stimulated new quality improvement strategies including Hospital and Physician Compare. It is possible that quality reporting may help promote standardization of care and reduce regional variation in costs.

With Regard to Cost Control

There has been a recent slowing of the rate of growth of healthcare cost increase [1]. Historically healthcare spending has risen as a share of GDP. Healthcare spending as a share of GDP remained relatively constant between 2009 and 2013; however there has been a recent increase beginning in 2014. As a share of GDP, total healthcare spending more than doubled from 1975 2013, increasing from 7.9 to 17.8%. Both private health insurance spending and Medicare spending more than tripled over that same time period, increasing from 1.8% to 5.9%, and from 1% to 3.6%, respectively, as a share of GDP [17] (Fig. 1.5).

The Congressional Budget Office projects a sustained slowing of the rate of Medicare expenditures to be less than 6% of the GDP [5] (Fig. 1.6). If this holds, it would further

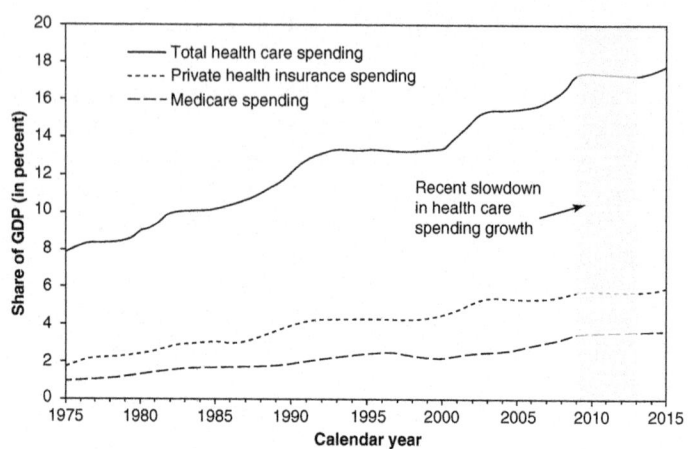

Note: GDP (gross domestic product).
Source: CMS Office of the Actuary, National Health Expenditure Accounts 2015.

FIGURE 1.5 Healthcare spending as a share of GDP

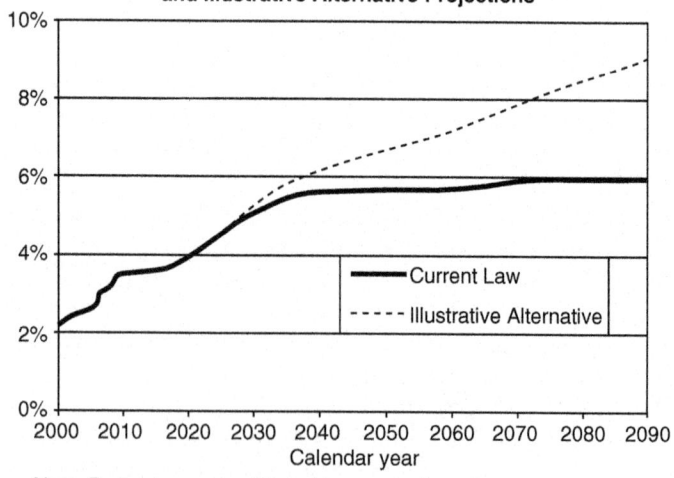

Note: Percentages are affected by economic cycles.

FIGURE 1.6 Medicare expenditures as a percentage of GDP [2]

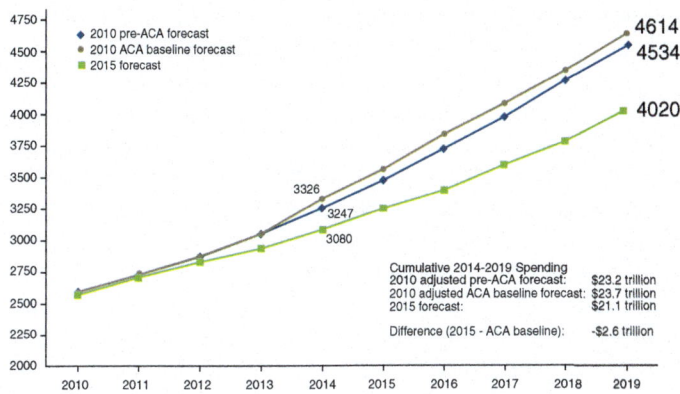

FIGURE 1.7 National health expenditure projections

extend the life of the Medicare Health Insurance Trust Fund without increasing beneficiary contributions or limiting benefits [3].

The Urban Institute projects a dramatic reduction in future national health expenditures based on value-based healthcare transformation and pay-for-quality performance related to the Medicare Access and Children's Health Insurance Program Reauthorization Act (MACRA) of 2015 [18] (Fig. 1.7). MACRA replaces Medicare's Sustainable Growth Rate formula (SGR) and is expected to be a potent lever driving physicians from fee-for-service to value-based-compliant practices (Chap. 2).

Will the Control of Healthcare Costs Be Lasting?

Is the slowing of the healthcare cost growth a reflection of quality metrics and structural change in healthcare? What is the contribution to healthcare spending of accepting more personal risk for health cost among employers and employees? Are there more far-reaching effects for accountability extending beyond health insurance premiums and co-pays? Will healthcare inflation continue to remain flat? These are all critical questions.

Unfortunately it appears that medical costs may be rising again after recent years of historic lows. Growth rates of medical spending from 2015 to 2017 have averaged 3.4% annually, up from the 0.9% in 2011–2013 [19]. In 2016, Medicare spending grew 3.6% and Medicaid spending grew 3.9% compared to total national health expenditures (NHE) which grew 4.3% [5]. Although the current growth rate is low in historical context, it exceeds the economy's growth as a whole, and healthcare costs are likely to be continually scrutinized with potential targeting of hospital, pharmaceutical, and physician reimbursement. While there may be savings associated with value-based purchasing, advanced alternative payment models (APMs) do not as yet make up the majority of the healthcare economy and it is unclear whether they will be sufficient to control healthcare spending in the long term.

If there has been a structural shift in healthcare spending associated with an increase in employer and consumer personal responsibility for health care, these factors may balance increased healthcare spending expected from a decline in the uninsured population and an improvement in the economy. This argument suggests that factors beyond the economy are contributing to sustain healthcare cost containment and that a return to fee-for-service volume-based health care will never occur. Value-based purchasing is, in all probability, here to stay.

Value-based healthcare purchasing is an external motivator for providers to reengineer healthcare delivery. Value-based purchasing is necessary for clinical quality improvement, but not sufficient to achieve this without population health management.

Incentives must also change as a prerequisite to healthcare delivery system transformation. Purchasers of health care must also implement the strategy of value-based purchasing. Effective healthcare services and high-performing healthcare providers are rewarded with improved reputations through public reporting, enhanced payments through differential reimbursements, and increased market share through purchaser, payer, and/or consumer selection. Purchasers, relying on quality, service, and cost, rather than cost alone, will catalyze the reengineering of health care toward a system of population health improvement and management and a value-driven system in which ever-increasing quality of care is achieved at the lowest possible cost [14].

If value-based purchasing continues, then pay-for-performance quality metrics follow. These ideas are not new. Numerous centers and institutes have proposed elements of value-based payment reform as a means to healthcare sustainability [20] (Fig. 1.8). There has also been a long history of CMS involvement since the 1970's with progressive in performance-based quality improvement strategy to improve health outcomes, improve standardization, reduce regional variation, and function as an efficient purchaser of healthcare resources on behalf of the public interest.

Table. Policy Comparisons

Policy[a]	Organization						
	Bipartisan Policy Center	Brookings Institution	The Commonwealth Fund	Kaiser Family Foundation[b]	National Coalition on Health Care	Partnership for Sustainable Health Care	Urban Institute
Value-based payment reform	✔	✔	✔	✔	✔	✔	✔
Value-based insurance design	✔	✔	✔	✔	✔	✔	✔
Efficient administration and markets							
Administrative/information technology	✔	✔	✔	✔	✔	✔	
Antitrust	✔	✔	✔	✔		✔	
Medical malpractice	✔	✔	✔	✔	✔	✔	
Evidence-based benefits	✔			✔	✔	✔	
Work force	✔	✔	✔		✔	✔	
Broad reforms							
Medicare structural reforms	✔		✔	✔			✔
Taxes	✔	✔		✔			✔
Caps	✔	✔		✔			

[a] Value-based payment reform: rewarding quality and better outcomes over volume of unit services. Value-based insurance design: benefit designs incentivizing patient choice ofh igher-quality treatments, clinicians, and hospitals and choice ofh ealthier lifestyles and adherence to effective treatment. Administrative/information technology: improvements that reduce costs. Antitrust: ensure healthy competition in local health care markets. Medical malpractice: liability policy improvement. Evidence-based benefits: paying for demonstrated clinical effectiveness. Work force: policies promoting provider efficiencies. Taxes: federal tax exemption changes enhancing insurance competition. Caps: total dollar limits, or targets with overspending consequences.

[b] Kaiser Family Foundation's January 2013 report presents an array of policy options without specific recommendations.

FIGURE 1.8 Healthcare policy recommendations. *Reproduced with permission from the publisher* [21]

Cost control will likely play a prominent role in future rounds of healthcare innovation and will be critical to sustaining coverage gains in the long term [22]. But much more needs to be done regarding issues of transparency, communication, coordination of health care across the continuum of care, education of healthcare providers, defining and measuring appropriate quality indicators, evaluating and rewarding risk, and partnering with consumers in achieving patient-centric goals of medical care.

References

1. World Health Organization, Geneva 2015. OCED Health Statistics 2015. https://www.oecd.org/unitedstates/Country-Note-UNITED%20STATES-OECD-Health-Statistics-2015.pdf. Accessed 17 Nov 2017.
2. Catlin AC, Cowan CA. History of health spending in the United States, 1960–2013. 2015. https://www.cms.gov/Research-Statistics-Data-and-Systems/Statistics-Trends-and-Reports/NationalHealthExpendData/Downloads/HistoricalNHEPaper.pdf. Accessed 17 Nov 2017.
3. The Boards of Trustees of the Federal Hospital Insurance and Federal Supplementary Medical Insurance Trust Funds. Annual Report of the Boards of Trustees of the Federal Hospital Insurance and Federal Supplementary Medical Insurance Trust Funds. 2016. https://www.cms.gov/Research-Statistics-Data-and-Systems/Statistics-Trends-and-Reports/ReportsTrustFunds/Downloads/TR2016.pdf. Accessed 24 Nov 2017.
4. Congressional Budget Office. Historical budget data, March 2016, and long-term budget projections, July 2016. https://www.cbo.gov/about/products/budget-economic-data. Accessed 10 Feb 2017.
5. Centers for Medicare Services and Medicaid Services National Health Expenditures Fact Sheet, December 6, 2017. https://www.cms.gov/research-statistics-data-and-systems/statistics-trends-and-reports/nationalhealthexpenddata/nhe-fact-sheet.html. Accessed 21 Dec 2017.
6. Butler SM. While replacing the ACA has republicans in ATC. JAMA. 2017;317:1514–5.

7. JAMA Infographic. JAMA. 2017;317:1516.
8. Martin AB, Hartman M, Washington B, Catlin A, Accounts National Health Expenditure Accounts Team. National health spending: master growth in 2015 has coverage expands and utilization increases. Health Aff. 2017;36:166–76.
9. Centers for Disease Control. National Center for Health Statistics. Health, United States; 2016. https://www.cdc.gov/nchs/fastats/health-expenditures.htm (overview- Table 94). Accessed 17 Nov 2017.
10. Emanuel EJ, Glickman A, Johnson D. Measuring the burden of health care costs on US families: the affordability index. JAMA. 2017;318:1863–4.
11. Kaiser HJ. Family Foundation. Employer health policy chart pack: Figure 5. 2017. https://www.kff.org/slideshow/2017-employer-health-benefits-chart-pack. Published September 2017. Accessed 24 Nov 2017.
12. Antos J, Capretta JC. Challenges in measuring the affordability of US health care. JAMA. 2017;318:1871–2.
13. Himmelstein D, Thorne D, Warren E, Woolhandler S. Medical bankruptcy in the United States, 2007: results of a national study. Am J Med. 2009;122(8):741–6.
14. National Business Council. Value – Based Purchasing. http://w.nbch.org/Value-based-Purchasing-A-Definition. Accessed 17 Nov 2017.
15. US Census Bureau. Health insurance coverage in the United States, 2016. Report Number P60-260. https://www.census.gov/library/publications/2017/demo/p60-260.html. Accessed 17 Nov 2017.
16. Centers for Medicare and Medicaid Services. Delivering Better Care at Lower Cost 9/16/14. https://www.cms.gov/Newsroom/MediaReleaseDatabase/Fact-sheets/2014-Fact-sheets-items/2014-09-16-2.html?DLPage=6&DLEntries=10&DLSort=0&DLSortDir=ascending. Accessed 17 Nov 2017.
17. Medicare Payment Advisory Commission. Data book: Beneficiaries dually eligible for Medicare and Medicaid – June 2017 MedPAC | MACPAC. http://www.medpac.gov/docs/default-source/data-book/jun17_databookentirereport_sec.pdf?sfvrsn=0. Accessed 17 Nov 2017.
18. McMorrow S, Holahan J. ACA implementation – monitoring and tracking. Executive summary: the widespread slowdown in health spending growth. Implications for future spending projections and the cost of the Affordable Care Act (RWJ/

Urban Institute). http://www.rwjf.org/content/dam/farm/reports/issue_briefs/2016/rwjf429930/subassets/rwjf429930_1. Accessed 17 Nov 2017.

19. Cutler DM. Rising medical cost meeting more rough times ahead. JAMA. 2017;318:508–9.
20. Lewin JC, Atkins GL, McNeely L. The elusive path to healthcare sustainability. JAMA. 2013;310:1669–70.
21. The Elusive Path to Health Care Sustainability. JAMA. 2013; 310(16):1669–70. doi:10.1001/jama.2013.280147.
22. Weiner J, Marks C, Polly M. Effects of the ACA on healthcare cost containment. University of Pennsylvania Leonard Davis Institute of health economics. 2017; 21(1). http://ldi.upenn.edu/sites/default/files/pdf/Effects%20of%20the%20ACA%20on%20Health%20Care%20Cost%20Containment%20-%20PennLDI%20ACA%20Impact%20Series.pdf. Accessed 17 Nov 2017.

Chapter 2
Quality Indicators, Outcomes, and Performance Pay

Abstract The history of the centers for Medicare Medicaid Services (CMS) involvement in quality improvement is long-standing. Linking performance metrics to payment is a powerful lever to stimulate healthcare improvement and maintenance of quality. This may also improve consistency and standardization of healthcare practices across regions.

Payment is a prime motivator for work effort. Linking performance metrics to payment is the new mantra for healthcare payment. Improvement and maintenance of quality and value-based purchasing are increasingly the norms for healthcare reimbursement. This pay-for-performance extends to healthcare institutions as well as to individual providers. It incentivizes global budgeting and bundling of procedures and services, limits government financial risk, and increases provider risk as well as potential for financial gain (two-tailed risk). Pay-for-performance encourages efficient resource management and a focus on outcomes, patient safety, and quality. Public reporting of quality measures increases accountability and transparency and promotes consistency and standardization of healthcare practices across regions.

The history of CMS involvement in quality improvement is long-standing. In recent years efforts by the Joint Commission, the Centers for Medicare and Medicaid Services (CMS), and

© Springer International Publishing AG, part of   15
Springer Nature 2018
J. S. Powers, *Value Driven Healthcare and Geriatric Medicine*,
https://doi.org/10.1007/978-3-319-77057-4_2

healthcare payers have focused on process measures to measure quality of care. Process measures can guide quality improvement efforts by assessing specific evidence-based processes of care within the control of healthcare providers.

Quality in Long-Term Care

Serious concerns about the quality of care in nursing homes have been reported for decades. In 1986, an Institute of Medicine (IOM), now called the National Academy of Medicine (NAM), report identified several problem areas with nursing home care, including staffing capacity, training, and supervision and made several recommendations regarding oversight and regulation to enhance nursing home standards, particularly those that received federal and state funding [1]. Subsequently, Congress enacted landmark legislation in the Omnibus Budget Reconciliation Act of 1987 (OBRA 87) that, among other provisions, established new minimum requirements for nursing homes eligible to receive Medicare or Medicaid payment, and put in place added enforcement systems. This linkage of quality performance as a condition of participation (and payment) was the first CMS entry into healthcare pay-for-performance measures. CMS mandated a comprehensive periodic assessment (minimum data set) where data quality metrics are compiled for each resident on admission, at quarterly intervals, and at the time of any significant change in condition. Nursing homes were also the first to experience public quality reporting, beginning with Nursing Home Compare in 1998. This nursing home care site, which is publicly accessible, provided information about size, staffing, services, and summary results of state inspections. In 2002 CMS introduced Quality Improvement Organizations (QIOs). The QIO focus included working with long-term care facilities to reduce the prevalence of pressure ulcers, the use of physical restraints, and the use of antipsychotic medications for managing behavior and individuals with dementia, reducing hospital readmissions within 30 days of discharge to post-acute care, and providing technical assistance in implementing Quality Assurance and Performance Improvement (QAPI), a data-driven, proactive approach to structure and promote quality improvement projects to enhance the quality of life, care, and services in nursing homes.

In 2008 the Five-Star rating system was initiated for long-term care. This rating system is composed of a composite score constructed from (1) the health survey measure derived from results of unannounced annual surveys by state surveyors, (2) a staffing measure dependent on the ratio of nursing staff to residents, and (3) performance rating on 18 separate quality-of-care measures. In 2015 these measures were recalibrated with respect to staffing hours per resident relative to the mix of resident care needs, and an increased emphasis on reduction of antipsychotic medication prevalence. Performance ratings of individual nursing homes are also being used as prerequisites to participate in advanced alternative payment healthcare models (APMs) such as next-generation account-able care organizations (ACOs). Changing benchmarks and quality-related conditions of participation are now increasingly common elements of healthcare contracts.

Quality in Home Health Care

Home Health Compare, another publicly accessible site, began in 2003 to evaluate home health services under the Consumer Assessment of Healthcare Providers and Systems (CAHPS). This model added quality measures to home care agency reporting requirements which were tied to the home health annual payment updates (Medicare APUs).

Quality in Hospital Care

Hospital Compare began in 2005. The Inpatient Quality Reporting Program currently consists of the following: (1) required reporting on 4 of 25 clinical quality measures such as venous thromboembolism prophylaxis, median time from emergency room arrival to departure, and home management plan-of-care document provided to patient or caregiver upon discharge; (2) required reporting on 24 claims-based measures such as 30-day readmission rate, excess days of care over benchmark, acute care measures for certain conditions such as acute myocardial infarction, congestive heart failure, pneumonia, and stroke, and inpatient mortality; and (3) HCAHPS survey of the patient's experience of inpatient care. This information is used for the annual payment update for the inpatient prospective payment system (Medicare IPPS−APU).

Quality Among Physicians

A pay-for-quality reporting system (PQRS) related to groups of physicians began in 2010. In 2012 quality reporting for groups of physicians was required in nine categories. Physician group practices can select from among numerous especially measure sets, including numbers of high-risk medications, blood pressure and diabetes control, breast and colorectal cancer screening, and immunization rates. In 2017 individual physician reporting became publicly available at the CMS Physician Compare website.

Physician payment has dramatically changed over time [2]. Previously Medicare payments to doctors were based on charges, but because of a high rate of medical inflation between 1980 and 1990, Congress determined that the professional payment rate for services would be determined by the resources necessary to perform them. This was reflected in the complexity weighting of Evaluation and Management (E&M) service codes, and annual increases for services were restricted based on the total volume of services delivered. These measures limited physician reimbursement to the overall Medicare budget. This slowed the rate of inflation somewhat, but in 1997 the sustainable growth rate (SGR) formula was instituted to force doctors to be more efficient. Utilization is the key factor driving SGR, which indexed physician payments relative to the gross domestic product (GDP) growth rate. Increased healthcare inflation relative to GDP therefore reduced physician reimbursement to maintain Medicare budget neutrality. However, when the SGR reduced physician payments, many physicians refused to see Medicare patients. To maintain Medicare access, a number of congressional interventions (termed doctor fix) to pay for a portion of the cuts were instituted; however the process became unsustainable. In 2015 the Medicare Access and Children's Health Insurance Program Reauthorization Act (MACRA) was passed with broad congressional support. MACRA replaces traditional Medicare fee for service with a two-track payment system.

Track 1 is the quality performance program (QPP), based on a merit-based incentive payment system (MIPS). This is Medicare's default payment track starting in 2019 to include an estimated 90% of US physicians not participating in advanced APMs. The first MIPS performance year is 2017 and will be used to determine payment adjustments, either a bonus or a penalty, that will be applied to Medicare Part B reimbursements to physicians beginning in 2019. Beginning in 2017, practices are scored across four categories: (1) cost, quality of resource utilization, and efficiency; (2) quality reporting measures; (3) advancing care information (ACI-electronic health records-EHR meaningful use); and (4) clinical practice quality improvement activity (QI) domains.

A composite performance score (CPS) sets annual incentives and penalties. Practices participating in MIPS reporting at least one quality measure, one practice improvement activity, and the required electronic health record measures in 2017 will avoid a negative payment adjustment in 2019. Those who report more than the minimum measures will receive higher scores and may receive a positive payment adjustment of up to 4% in 2019. Only clinicians reporting no measures or activities in 2017 will receive a negative adjustment (maximum negative adjustment 4% starting in 2019).

Clinicians are being assessed by comparing a CPS to a threshold score set by CMS. Practices must now report six quality measures from over 300 approved measures, as appropriate to their individual healthcare system or specialty. The weights of the CPS elements will change over time with increasing weight of the cost variable and decreasing weight of the quality reporting measures. The ACI and QI domain weights will remain stable. Practices, identified by group billing ID, are left to make strategic decisions to choose quality reporting measures and practice quality improvement activities in order to perform well. CMS has invited medical specialty societies to develop quality indicators appropriate to specialty practices [3].

Cost will be a major contributor to the CPS, set at 10% beginning in 2020, and rising to 30% in 2021 and forward (Table 2.1). Cost considers the relationship of the physician to the patient and needs to be attributed appropriately to equitably adjust for cost among practitioners. CMS is implementing a value-based modifier system that will assign all Medicare A and B expenses to each practitioner responsible for such costs. Managing patients with multiple clinical conditions and transitional care management requires dedicated office staff, team-based care, and significant non-face-to-face time. Estimates of cost are critical to physician buy-in and there is a need to better align to the service provided than have previous E&M service codes, and disease-state criteria. Additionally,

TABLE 2.1 MIPS CPS scoring [4]

CPS category	2017–2019	2020	2021 (and subsequent years)
Cost	0	10%	30%
Quality measures	60%	50%	30%
ACI	25%	25%	25%
QI	15%	15%	15%

MIPS merit-based incentive payment system, *CPS* composite performance score, *ACI* advancing care information (EMR), *QI* practice quality improvement activities the determination of triggers for episodes of care, or groupings of episodes of care for chronic disease models, is important for appropriate risk adjustment and attributed cost cross the healthcare continuum. CMS has encouraged medical societies to propose chronic disease models and sets of measures, and to validate a definition of continuous relationship with the patient to help structure cost factors. The American Geriatrics Society has developed position statements on goals of care and advance care planning, complex care management, coordination of care, care transitions, caregiver support, and standards for skilled nursing facility care, home-based care, medication reconciliation post-discharge, care of urinary incontinence, fall risk assessment, use of high-risk medications in elderly, and dementia and cognitive assessment. Operationalizing the measurement, reporting, and cost attributes of these conditions continues, with contributions from medical societies including the American College of Physicians, the American Medical Association, and other specialty societies. Beginning in 2017, CMS has also begun to reduce the 15% increased payment (facility fee) to hospital-owned outpatient departments as part of the site neutrality provision of the 2015 Bipartisan Budget Act.

Track 2 includes advanced alternative payment models (APMs). Advanced APMs include certain qualifying models as determined by CMS such as next-generation ACOs, Bundled Payment Care Initiatives (BCPIs), Comprehensive Primary Care Plus (CPC+), and Medicare Track 2 and 3 Shared Savings Programs (MSSPs). Practices in advanced APMs are exempt from MIPS reporting requirements, incentives, and penalties. Practitioners are being encouraged to develop and participate in these new models of care; however only approximately 10% of physicians are expected to be participating in advanced APMs as of 2019. Practices in advanced APMs receive a 5% annual payment bonus in Medicare Part B payment from 2019 to 2024 [5–7]. However all APMs inherently have significant startup costs and certain advanced APMs entail acceptance of downside risk.

MIPS bonuses are structured as rate increases related to Medicare Part B services. This could incentivize providers to deliver higher cost services. The use of national quality benchmarks tends to make clinical performance influenced by the population of patients served rather than the quality of care. Without risk adjustment to account for patient population differences, MIPS could transfer resources to providers serving lower risk patients, and incentivizes favorable selection processes to obtain lower risk patients. Quality scoring permits providers to select from a limited number of measures, possibly diluting the effect of MIPS in achieving a meaningful effect with respect to improving quality of care. CMS is driving providers towards advanced APMs designed with stronger incentives to decrease spending and increase quality of care. MIPS could however be improved by restructuring bonuses as fixed per-beneficiary payments referenced to quality improvement adjusted to prior performance [8].

Compensating physicians under value-based care models challenges physicians' desire for clinical autonomy. Value-based compensation may be viewed as subjective, with performance measures based on factors outside physician's direct control such as staff and patient behaviors which impact overall outcomes. As the industry transitions to value-based payments, some compensation still needs to be tied to productivity so that physicians can directly impact performance. Whichever quality metrics are tied to financial incentives, they need to be consistent with the group's mission and values and also enforce strategic objectives [9].

If pay for value is to stimulate the delivery of better health and better results for all then we must measure what matters most, utilizing consistent core metrics to sharpen and focus on performance. We must accelerate the acquisition of real-world evidence and facilitate the clinician's capability to derive evidence from each care experience. This is a huge challenge for refinement of EHR systems to provide feedback to clinicians and for development of big data management capabilities.

Quality in Hospital Care

In 1972 the Title XI Amendment of the Social Security Act created Professional Standards Review Organizations (PSROs). These physician-sponsored organizations used local physicians to evaluate cases to determine medical necessity for hospital care. They also performed retrospective utilization review of hospital admissions and length of stay [10]. The Peer Review Improvement Act of 1982 transformed the PSROs into peer review organizations (PROs). The focus shifted from retrospective review of individual providers to prospectively evaluating practice patterns and using physician content expertise to guide quality improvement at institutional and regional levels. CMS expanded the healthcare quality improvement program in 1995 using the PROs as part of a comprehensive program to enhance quality improvement work across the Medicare and Medicaid programs. CMS renamed the PROs as Quality Improvement Organizations (QIOs) in 2002 to reflect Medicare's evolving emphasis on improving clinical quality of care. The QIOs were very important in benchmarking and standardizing quality indicators for hospital, long-term care, home and community-based care, and outpatient settings.

As a result of CMS' increasing emphasis on quality, there were national improvements in 20 out of 22 indicators for Medicare fee-for-service care between 1998 and 2001, including 19.9% for outpatient indicators and 11.9% for inpatient indicators. Improvement was most marked in states with the lowest quality performance indicators [11]. Individual quality indicators are shown in Table 2.2. Similarly hospitals that participate in QIO activities tend to have higher quality indicators than hospitals that do not participate [12].

Standardization of healthcare processes enhances organizational oversight and may contribute to improved quality of care. Beginning in 2014, QIOs began to collaborate as regional multistate entities, Quality Innovation Networks (QIN-QIOs) to share best practices, and to enlarge the scope of influence to involve all healthcare practices [13].

TABLE 2.2 CMS QIO quality indicators (2000)

Inpatient

Acute myocardial infarction

- Administration of aspirin within 24 h of admission
- Aspirin prescribed at discharge
- Administration of beta-blocker within 24 h of patient admission
- Beta-blocker prescribed at discharge
- ACE inhibitors prescribed at discharge (ejection fraction less than 40%)
- Smoking cessation counseling given during hospitalization
- Time to angioplasty (minutes)
- Time to thrombolytic therapy (minutes)

Heart failure

- Evaluation of ejection fraction
- ACE inhibitors prescribed at discharge (ejection fraction less than 40%)

Stroke

- Warfarin prescribed for patients with atrial fibrillation
- Antithrombotic prescribed at discharge (stroke or TIA)
- Avoidance of sublingual nifedipine for patients with acute stroke

Pneumonia

- Antibiotic within 8 h of arrival at hospital; antibiotic consistent with current recommendations
- Blood culture drawn (if done) before antibiotic given
- Patient screened for and given influenza vaccine
- Patient screened for and given pneumococcal vaccine

TABLE 2.2 (continued)

Any setting

Pneumonia

- Influenza immunization every year

- Pneumococcal immunization at least once

Breast cancer

- Mammogram at least every 2 years

Diabetes

- Hemoglobin A_{1c} at least yearly

- Diabetic eye exam at least every 2 years

- Lipid profile at least every 2 years

Quality Process Measures and Outcome Measures

The Joint Commission proposes that process measures should meet four criteria: (1) there should be a strong evidence base showing that the care process leads to improved clinical outcomes, (2) the process measure must accurately capture whether the care process has been provided, (3) the process measure must be closely linked to the outcome with few intervening processes, and (4) implementation of the measurements should have little or no chance of producing unintended adverse consequences [14].

Federal public reporting and payment programs are now focusing less on measuring processes and more on measuring outcomes such as 30-day readmission rates and mortality, and patient-reported outcome measures (PROMs) such as changes in pain and physical functioning. Outcome measures are of the greatest interest to consumers and payers as they help quantify the end results of health care. However, the criteria for assessing whether outcome measures are accurate and valid enough to use for public reporting, payment, and accreditation are not well defined. Additionally, outcome measures can be greatly influenced by characteristics of the patient population across providers.

In order for a valid process–outcome link to exist, four additional criteria should be met: (1) strong evidence should exist that good medical care leads to improvement in the outcome within the time period for the measure, (2) the outcome should be measurable with a high degree of precision, (3) the risk adjustment methodology should include and accurately measure the risk factors most strongly associated with the outcome, and (4) implementation of the outcome measure must have little chance of causing adverse consequences [15] (Table 2.3).

Currently data linking good medical care to improvement in outcome may not exist in order to determine whether the effect of good medical care on outcomes is great enough for the measure to be used for accountability. The use of claims data can be problematic especially if conditions present on admission, or secondary diagnoses, are not accounted for. Measuring outcomes across providers must be uniform in order to avoid bias in performance rates. Accurate measurement of PROMs is challenging because of the difficulty in collecting data directly from patients and assuring an adequate response rate. Almost

TABLE 2.3 Criteria for accountability measures address health outcomes [15]

1. Strong evidence should exist that good medical care leads to improvement in the outcome within the time period for the measure

2. The outcome should be measurable with a high degree of precision

3. The risk adjustment methodology should include and accurately measure the risk factors most strongly associated with the outcome

4. Implementation of the outcome measure must have little chance of causing adverse consequences

all outcome measures will require risk adjustment to account for differences in the severity of the patient's illness, comorbid conditions, physiological state, and socioeconomic status that are not under the provider's control. The prevalence of these risk factors for the outcome may vary across providers reflective of the different populations that they serve. Additionally outcome measures should be avoided if they promote unintended consequences with undesirable practice changes driven by incentives rather than by patient outcomes [15].

An assessment of 10 of the approximately 40 outcome measures used and public reporting and payment programs is displayed in Table 2.4. Concerns identified suggest that mortality measures fare poorly, claims-based risk adjustment methodology is unclear, and surveillance bias can greatly influence outcome measurements.

The identification and use of appropriate outcome measures to drive quality improvement require extreme care. Solid evidence for a link between clinical interventions and outcomes is a cornerstone of a meaningful measure and is required for endorsement by the National Quality Forum (NQF). There is a great deal of work necessary to verify the accuracy of submitted quality data. We also need better clinical and social data for risk assessment to enable stratification and adjustment, and to direct targeted improvement. Feedback from providers and consumers is critical to support a learning healthcare system which monitors the effect of measurement for adverse consequences as well as improved clinical outcomes [16].

There are also costs involved in quality measurements. These may include fixed costs associated with implementing a quality measurement infrastructure, and these can be born at multiple levels such as government, hospitals, or practices. Measures requiring dedicated data collection such as patient-reported outcome surveys (PROMs) are particularly costly. Better understanding of the cost of measures would help inform decisions about which measures to use as well as guide future development of high-value market measures to maximize benefit and minimize the use of finite quality measurement resources [17].

TABLE 2.4 Outcome measures and assessments of whether they meet the proposed accountability criteria [15]. Reproduced with permission of the publisher

Topic	Measurement method	Outcome	Criterion 1		Criterion 2	Criterion 3		Criterion 4
			Evidence that good care improves the outcome	Appropriate measurement period	Precise outcome measurement	Key risk factors included	Precise risk factor measurement	Low chance of adverse consequences
COPD	Claims	30-d mortality	Yes, limited[a]	No	Yes	No[b]	No	Yes
Heart failure	Claims	30 d mortality	Yet	No[c]	Yes	No[d]	NA[e]	Yes
Stroke	Claims	30-d mortality	No	No	Yes	No	No	No
Pneumonia	Claims	30-d mortality	Yes	Yes	No	No	No	Yes
Coronary artery bypass grafting[f]	–	30-d mortality	Yes	Yes	Yes	Yes	Yes	Yes[g]
NSQIP surgical site infection	Chart	Infection within 30 d	Yes	Yes	Yes	Yes	Yes	Yes[h]
NHSN central line-associated bloodstream infection	Chart	New bloodstream infection after central line placement	Yes	Yes	Probably[i]	Yes	Yes	Yes

VTE after surgery	Claims	New VTE during hospitalization	Yes	Yes	No[j]	No	NA[e]	No
Change in physical function and pain after joint replacement	Patient survey	Change in measure during 12 mo after surgery	Yes	Yes	Yes if high response rate	Yes	Yes	Yes[g]
HCAHPS	Patient survey	Rating of experience of care during hospital stay	Yes	Yes	Unclear because of low response rate	Yes	Yes	Uncertain

COPD chronic obstructive pulmonary disease, *HCAHPS* hospital consumer assessment of healthcare providers and systems, *NA* not applicable, *NHSN* National healthcare safety network, *NSQIP* National surgical quality improvement project, *VTE* venous thromboembolism

[a] The only treatment shown to affect mortality for COPD is home oxygen therapy for patients with resting hypoxemia during baseline health (i.e., not during an exacerbation). Most patients hospitalized with COPD do not have baseline hypoxemia

[b] Claims data do not capture such risk factors as FEV_1 and current smoking status

TABLE 2.4 (continued)

[c] In the major studies of heart failure treatment, mortality was examined over a much longer period than 30 d. However, differences in 30-d mortality could be detected between hospitals with very poor and excellent adherence to several recommended treatments

[d] Claims data do not capture left ventricular ejection fraction and baseline physical functioning (e.g., New York Heart Association classification)

[e] If key risk factors are not included, whether others are measured precisely does not matter

[f] We show assessments based on the New York State Cardiac Surgery Reporting System and the Society of Thoracic Surgeons National Database

[g] Concerns exist regarding whether these outcome measures might cause surgeons to be less likely to operate on more severely ill patients, even though such patients may greatly benefit from the procedures. However, evidence that this potential problem actually occurs in practice is limited

[h] Monitoring surgical site infections might lead to overuse of antibiotics. Although evidence that this actually occurs in practice is lacking, continued monitoring of this potential problem is needed

[i] Concerns were raised recently that hospitals are not adhering to NHSN protocols and that the accuracy of this measure may have diminished

[j] Studies suggest that rates of VTE are highly subject to surveillance bias, which probably explains why institutions with higher rates of prophylaxis have higher VTE rates

References

1. National Academies of Science Engineering and Medicine. Improving the quality of care in nursing homes. 1986. http://www.nationalacademies.org/hmd/Reports/1986/Improving-the-Quality-of-Care-in-Nursing-Homes.aspx. Accessed 17 Nov 2017.

2. Mitchell E. Population-based payment models: overcoming barriers, accelerating adoption. May 16, 2016. https://hcp-lan.org/2016/05/pbp-models-overcoming-barriers-accelerating-adoption/. Accessed 17 Nov 2017.

3. Institute of Medicine. Vital signs: core metrics for health and health care progress. Washington, DC: National Academies Press; 2015.

4. Office of the Federal Register. Medicare Program; Merit-based Incentive Payment System (MIPS) and Alternative Payment Model (APM) incentive under the physician fee schedule, and criteria for physician-focused payment models, 42 CFR Parts 414 and 495. Published in the Federal Register 11/4/16: https://www.federalregister.gov/documents/2016/11/04/2016-25240/medicare-program-merit-based-incentive-payment-system-mips-and-alternative-payment-model-apm. Accessed 17 Nov 2017.

5. Centers for Medicare & Medicaid Services. Quality payment programs. Executive summary. https://qpp.cms.gov/docs/QPP_Executive_Summary_of_Final_Rule.pdf. Accessed 17 Nov 2017.

6. Unroe KT, Hollmann PA, Goldstein AC, Maline ML. Medicare access and CHIP reauthorization intact: what do geriatrics healthcare professionals need to know about the quality payment program? JAGS. 2017;65:674–9.

7. American College of Physicians. Comment: Medicare Program; Merit-Based Incentive Payment System (MIPS) and Alternative Payment Model (APM) Incentive under the Physician fee schedule, and criteria for physician-focused payment models [CMS-5517-FC]. https://www.acponline.org/acp_policy/letters/avp_comment_letter_to_cms_on_macra_final_rule_2016.pdf. Accessed 17 Nov 2017.

8. McWilliams JM. MACRA: big fix or big problem? Ann Intern Med. 2017;167:122–4.

9. Gagliano N. Satisfaction vs burnout. Value-based strategies that motivate. Group Pract J. 2017:15–17.

10. Medicare's Quality Improvement Organization program: Maximizing potential. Pathways to healthcare. http://www.nap.edu/catalog/11604.html. Accessed 17 Nov 2017.

11. Jencks SF, Huff ED, Cuerdon T. Change in the quality of care delivered to Medicare beneficiaries, 1998–1999 to 2000–2001. JAMA. 2003;289:305–12.
12. Snyder C, Anderson G. Do quality improvement organizations improve the quality of hospital care for Medicare beneficiaries? JAMA. 2005;293:2900–7.
13. Mims AD, Pederson JC, Gold JA. Healthcare changes and the affordable care act: a physician call to action quality improvement organizations. In: Powers JS, editor. Healthcare changes and the affordable care act. Switzerland: Springer International Publishing; 2015. p. 13–31.
14. Chassin MR, Loeb JM, Schmaltz SP, Wachter RM. Accountability measures–using measurement to promote quality improvement. N Engl J Med. 2010;363:683–8.
15. Baker DW, Chassin MR. Holding providers accountable for healthcare outcomes. Ann Intern Med. 2017;167:418–23.
16. Burstin H, Qaseem A. Moving to measures that matter and motivate change. Ann Intern Med. 2017;167:442–3.
17. Schuster MA, Oronata SE, Meltzer DO. Measuring the cost of quality measurement: a missing link in quality strategy. JAMA. 2017;318:1219–20.

Chapter 3
Are the Drivers of Healthcare Change Changing Healthcare Outcomes?

Abstract The Centers for Medicare and Medicaid Services (CMS) measures success defined as improving the patient's experience of care within the National Academy of Medicine's six aims for healthcare improvement: safety, effectiveness, patient centeredness, timeliness, efficiency, and equity. Better health is defined as increasing the overall health of populations. Improved quality of care could reduce overall healthcare cost and the patient's experience of care.

Forces of Change

Outcome measures, pay-for-performance, and external regulations can be strong levers for change. These factors, combined with other important developments such as the transparency of publicly accessed Physician Compare and Maintenance of Certification (MOC) data, have the potential to create major changes in physician behavior. Maintenance of certification and quality metrics may indeed become new conditions of employment, licensure, reimbursement, and even medical liability coverage.

The forces of value-based purchasing have created a sea change in the marketplace regarding reimbursement for medical services. We are seeing the demise of fee-for-service (FFS) for practically all lines of healthcare coverage. Professional

© Springer International Publishing AG, part of   33
Springer Nature 2018
J. S. Powers, *Value Driven Healthcare and Geriatric Medicine*,
https://doi.org/10.1007/978-3-319-77057-4_3

societies need to help clinicians and practices understand and prepare for the new world of value-based reimbursement.

There is a belief that standardization, reducing variation, and quality reporting measures will drive quality improvement. The American College of Physicians supports quality improvement as part of professionalism with three commitments linking professionalism with the public's health: (1) improving the quality of care, (2) improving access to care, and (3) just distribution of resources. Given the burden that healthcare costs impose on society and the magnitude of inefficiency in the current system, the federal government should continue to press forward with payment and delivery reforms. The measure of their success will be whether health care improves and healthcare cost growth slows for the US population overall (Table 3.1) [1].

Value-based care is also supported by the triple aims of the Institute of Medicine, now called the National Academy of Medicine (NAM), which are (1) improved care experience for the patient, (2) improved quality of care, and (3) cost-effective care, including cost avoidance. How is it possible to harness the population demands for primary care, continuity of care, quality of care, and transparency in order to create value for all? [2].

TABLE 3.1 CMS measures of success

1. Better health care defined as improving the patient's experience of care within the Institute of Medicine's six aims for healthcare improvement: safety, effectiveness, patient centeredness, timeliness, efficiency, and equity

2. Better health by keeping patients well so they can do what they want to do. Increasing the overall health of populations: addressing behavioral risk factors, and focusing on preventive care

3. Reduced costs by lowering the total cost of care will improve quality resulting in reduced expenditures for Medicare, Medicaid, and Children's Health Insurance Program beneficiaries (CHIP)

Many call for more research and evidence on payment reforms and healthcare restructuring. But stakeholders interpret data differently, demonstrating a divide over an acceptable threshold of evidence for action. Academic medical centers prize rigorous high-quality evidence to minimize the possibility that results are due to random chance or other confounding factors. The evaluation of value-based purchasing which is occurring during the course of its evolution can complicate interpretation of results. In contrast the business community prioritizes speed and timely information. A healthcare innovation may require months or years before it can be fully evaluated and scaled to larger populations. Healthcare payers may therefore pilot and expand a payment model well before there is definite evidence of its success — although this can be risky. Business has therefore often used rapid-cycle longitudinal designs to evaluate reforms.

The CMS Office of the Actuary has adopted a middle-ground approach for determining whether to scale a pilot healthcare innovation. CMS usually pilots the innovation first with a limited number of providers or locations as a demonstration to gather evidence about performance. CMS must certify that the evidence indicates that the innovation would reduce cost or at least have a budget-neutral effect on program spending so that CMS does not have to wait for years for the results of randomized controlled studies. Similarly, legislative action is often taken if the totality of the evidence shows improvement. CMS routinely provides quarterly feedbacks to its payment and model participants and publishes public reports on a model's performance.

Implementation science can be a potential catalyst for delivery system review. There is a growing interest in patient involvement in healthcare innovations recognizing that the increasing burden of chronic illness in the population cannot be addressed without engaging patients and their caregivers in effective self-care. There is a great need to better align treatment choices with patients' well-informed preferences and values to permit shared decision-making between patients and providers. A comprehensive framework such as implementation science is needed to identify the ways with which patient engagement strategies can be adopted and spread throughout the healthcare system. We must support and adapt an existing inpatient-driven regulatory framework with a blend of real-world and scientific clinical trial evidence. We need key real-world data such as downstream clinical information and patient-reported outcomes in order to measure real progress in healthcare outcomes [3]. Quality reporting drives new electronic health record (EHR) technology such as dashboards providing real-time reporting for providers. Public reporting of quality indicators increases transparency and influences the reputation, or public's perception of healthcare institutions and individual providers. This focus on outcomes, driven by value-based purchasing, could theoretically improve quality and the patient's experience of care.

Evidence for Quality Improvement

While only an estimated 10–15% of providers are presently in advanced alternative payment models (APMs), there is increasing evidence that health outcome quality and value have improved with quality reporting in several significant areas. Passage of the Hospital Readmissions Reduction Program (HRRP) required CMS to reduce payments to hospitals with higher-than-expected readmission rates for targeted conditions, including heart failure, acute myocardial infarction, and pneumonia. Hospitals were provided readmission performance data relative to peers beginning in 2009, with financial penalties beginning in 2012. Thirty-day readmission rates for these three conditions collectively declined from 21.5 to 17.8% between 2007 and 2015 [4]. Strategies designed to lower readmissions through improved inpatient [5], transitional care [6–8], and post-acute care [9, 10] and communication among physicians and healthcare professionals across care settings may have reduced both readmission and mortality rates following hospitalization. Reductions in hospital 30-day readmission rates are also correlated with reductions in hospital 30-day mortality rates after discharge suggesting that there has been no increase in mortality associated with reduced rehospitalization rates [11].

Between 2013 and 2017 preventable hospitalizations decreased 7%, from 53.8 to 49.9 discharges per 1000 Medicare enrollees. Hospital readmissions decreased 7% during the same time period from 15.9 to 14.8% of hospitalized Medicare enrollees. Hospital laboratory testing decreased 30%, from 30.1 to 21%, and hospice care use increased 42%, from 37.7 to 52% of chronically ill Medicare decedents aged 65 years and older. ICU use in the last 6 months of life decreased 9%, from 15.2 to 13.8% of Medicare decedents aged 65 years and older. The hip fracture hospitalization rate likewise decreased 21%, from 7.3 to 5.8 hospitalizations per 1000 Medicare enrollees [12].

The 30-day readmission for myocardial infarction, heart failure, and pneumonia decreased more rapidly than before the HRRP and improvement was most marked for hospitals with the highest readmission rate [13]. In 2017, 79% of eligible hospitals were penalized by CMS with an average penalty of 0.74% (max 3%) of Medicare inpatient payments [14]. However there has been a slowing of improvements in inpatient mortality for pneumonia, acute myocardial infarction, and congestive heart failure during the same period [15, 16]. These data deserve further study and question whether a floor for mortality has been reached or whether resources have been diverted away from mortality towards decreased hospital readmissions, given lower incentives for mortality quality improvement than 30-day readmission rates under the hospital value-based purchasing program [17]. Readmission reductions for targeted conditions also appear to be accompanied by lower readmission rates for other conditions [18]. Accountable care organizations (ACOs) have shown have shown an overall improvement in meeting quality indicators, increasing composite scores from 70 to 84% [19].

Bundled Payments for Care Improvement (BPCI) is a voluntary program phased in between 2013 and 2015 in which some 1400 organizations are currently participating. The BPCI initiative is comprised of four broadly defined models of care, which link payments for the multiple services beneficiaries receive during an episode of care. There are presently some 48 bundles from which participants are able to choose [20]. Under the initiative, organizations enter into payment arrangements that include financial and performance accountability for episodes of care. The model entails risk bearing if total cost for the episode exceeds the target price, but participating organizations also share some portion of the cost savings with CMS.

ACOs are provided a prospective payment to manage a local population of Medicare patients selected by CMS. ACOs have populations assigned by CMS to equitably distribute risk within patient populations. There is a gradual phase-in of risk over a 3-year period with an initial shared savings, subsequently adding downside (loss) risk with an increased incentive for shared profits. An evaluation of hospital participation in voluntary value-based models of care which included meaningful use of electronic health records, Bundled Payment for Care Initiative episode-based payment program (BPCI), or the Pioneer and shared savings ACO programs was associated with greater reductions in 30-day readmissions for acute myocardial infarction, heart failure, and pneumonia compared to hospitals that did not participate in these programs. Participation in multiple programs led to greater reductions in 30-day readmissions [21]. In the first 2 years of the Pioneer ACO model, beneficiaries aligned with Pioneer ACOs, as compared to general Medicare fee-for-service beneficiaries, exhibited smaller increases in total Medicare expenditures with some reductions in utilization of different health services, with little difference in patient-related experience [22].

In the home health arena, the average risk-adjusted rate of hospitalization for home care patients decreased in recent years from a high of 28.8% in 2008 but still remains over 25% [23].

Skilled nursing facilities (SNF) have improved on some measures but not others from 2011 to 2015. Rates of risk-adjusted community discharges and potentially avoidable readmissions during the SNF stay improved between 2011 and 2015. The 13 potentially avoidable conditions include congestive heart failure, electrolyte imbalance/dehydration, respiratory infection, sepsis, urinary tract or kidney infection, hypoglycemia or diabetic complications, anticoagulant complications, fractures and musculoskeletal injuries, acute delirium, adverse drug reactions, cellulitis/infections, pressure ulcers, and abnormal blood pressure. A greater share of beneficiaries was discharged to the community (38.8% compared with 33.2%). During the same period, fewer beneficiaries were readmitted to acute care hospitals during the SNF stay (10.4% compared with 12.4%) or in the 30 days after discharge from the SNF (5% compared with 5.9%) [23]. Risk-adjusted measures of change in functional status were essentially unchanged between 2011 and 2015. These functional mobility measures are composites of the patient's abilities in bed mobility, transfer, and ambulation. The rate of improvement in mobility includes the share of stays with improvement in one, two, or three activities of daily living: bed mobility, transfer, and ambulation.

There is evidence that Nursing Home Compare, a website that publicly reports quality measures on nursing homes, has been influential in driving reduction of restraints as well as antipsychotic use prevalence. There have been long-standing concerns about the safety and efficacy of antipsychotic agents used to treat behavioral symptoms of dementia. The Centers for Medicare and Meducaid Services launched the National Partnership to Improve Dementia Care in Nursing Homes in 2012, with a focus on protecting residents from being prescribed antipsychotic medications unless there is a valid, clinical indication and a systemic process to evaluate each individual's need. In 2015, CMS also added the prevalence of nursing home residents receiving antipsychotics to the Five-Star Quality Rating System for nursing homes. By the end of 2016, the percentage of long-term residents receiving antipsychotic therapy had decreased from 24 to 16%. (Fig. 3.1) To achieve its objective of reducing antipsychotic medication utilization, CMS endorsed five strategies:

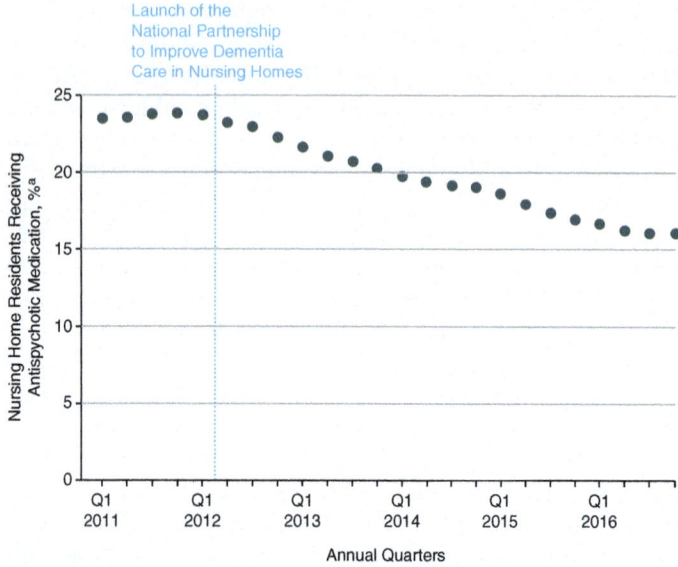

FIGURE 3.1 Percentage of long-term nursing home residents receiving antipsychotic medication, 2011–2016 [24]. Reproduced with permission from the publisher

(1) engaging stakeholders, (2) creating and disseminating educational resources, (3) public reporting of antipsychotic prevalence in nursing homes as a quality measure, (4) enhancing guidance and training of state surveyors, and (5) increasing enforcement of regulations with civil monetary penalties for noncompliance [24].

Pay-for-performance programs may be associated with improved processes of care in ambulatory settings but consistently positive associations with improved health problems have not been demonstrated in any setting [25]. Medicare advantage plans do better on some measures like preventive care. Counties with greater Medicare advantage penetration appear to improve traditional Medicare's performance [26]. Medicare advantage plans however have lower patient satisfaction scores among sicker members [27]. Quality measures for Medicare Advantage health maintenance organizations

(HMOs) have shown that quality measures were generally stable between 2014 and 2016. These measures included (1) the Healthcare Effectiveness Data and Information Set (Hedis®) administrative measures: osteoporosis management and rheumatoid arthritis management; (2) Hedis® Hybrid Measures: body mass index documentation, colorectal cancer screening, controlling blood pressure, eye exam to check for damage from diabetes, kidney function testing for members with diabetes, and diabetics not controlling blood sugar; (3) measures from the Health Outcome Survey (HOS®): advising physical activity and reducing the risk of falling; (4) other measures based on HOS®: improving or maintaining physical health, and improving or maintaining mental health; and (5) measures from the Consumer Assessment of Healthcare Providers and Systems (CAHPS®): annual flu vaccine, ease of getting needed care and seeing specialists, getting appointments in care quickly, and overall rating of quality and health care quality [23].

In 2015 the Medicare Access and Children's Health Insurance Program Reauthorization Act (MACRA) was passed with broad congressional support. MACRA replaces traditional Medicare fee for service with a two track payment system. Track 1 is the quality performance program (QPP), based on a merit-based incentive payment system (MIPS). Track 2 includes advanced alternative payment models (APMs) such as accountable care organizations (ACOs), patient-centered medical homes, and bundled payment models. Practices in APMs are exempt from MIPS reporting requirements, incentives, and penalties. Pay for performance continues to develop but it will take years to understand and refine the quality metrics. To date the relationship between pay for performance, performance incentives, and effectiveness in promoting physician behavior change has not been empirically studied. In general simple choices and immediate feedback are generally more influential than complex choices and delayed feedback to providers. Yet the merit-based incentive payment system (MIPS) is an elaborate policy that applies incentives 2 years after the care is provided. Additionally, social and medical risk adjustment may be necessary for some practice populations. During the first year of the Medicare physician value-based payment modifier program, physician practices that serve more socially high-risk patients had lower quality and lower costs and practices that serve more medically high-risk patients had lower quality and higher costs [28, 29]. See Chap. 2 for a more detailed explanation of MIPS.

Closely associated with pay-for-performance is the concept of high-value care: cost-conscious care which eliminates unsafe and low-value services that generate expenses with potential harm or no benefit to the patient. The Choosing Wisely Campaign, developed by the American Board of Internal Medicine Foundation, is a program to find approaches to remove waste and ineffective care from our healthcare system. Specialty societies have also stepped up to the plate. Contributions from 70 medical and surgical specialty organizations have identified over 300 areas of ineffective clinical care, resulting in new guidelines for care. Early data suggest that the campaign has had some success in moving the standard of care by promoting the adoption of some practices and discontinuation of ineffective or wasteful practices [30].

Measures of success in terms of healthcare process and outcomes include target measures for chronic illness, preventive care services such as immunizations and screening, and appropriate use of resources. Some of these outcomes are reflected in claims data, and other quality indicators are obtained from the electronic health record (EHR). The emphasis on outcome measures as part of value-driven health care makes quality a priority focus for the healthcare system, the provider, and ultimately the patient. Incentivizing quality can improve process measures rather quickly with savings on claims spending reflecting meaningful behavior change.

Increasing integration among physicians and hospitals affords delivery systems more market power to bargain for prices and spending targets. Conversely, private payers might respond by enhancing their own market power through acquisition and consolidation. There is potential for coordination between public and private payers to create a favorable balance between regulatory and market-based approaches to slow spending. Such coordinated efforts may also help physicians and hospitals disseminate new delivery system models to patients across different payers [31].

The focus on quality and cost-effectiveness is pervasive in its effects. Practices and hospitals are rushing to adopt reporting-compliant EHR capabilities, in part sparked by financial incentives under EHR Incentive Programs. CMS' hope is that sustained support of real-time provision of data and practice feedback will improve the quality of care.

Example: Adoption of an Electronic Health Record (EHR) Reporting-Compliant System

Performance metrics are powerful levers to drive quality and treatment data reporting. Our university hospital developed a homegrown EHR and utilized it successfully since the 1990s. Initially ahead of its time, it became increasingly evident that it was unable to respond to the external environment and demands required by value-based purchasing. It was unable to create dashboards and was inefficient in collecting quality reporting data and supporting primary care processes. Additionally it was incapable of communication with other EHRs, even within the institution. Over the years it had been continuously updated to respond to new physician order sets; however many components were not linked including nurses' notes and rehabilitation treatments. The university ultimately adopted a new commercial system after 2 years of deliberation driven mainly by threat of Medicare penalties for noncompliance in reporting quality indicators, and in order to maintain timely and appropriate billing, coding, and reimbursement for the institution. The new system now provides point-of-care dashboards and quarterly data at the provider level, structured notes, medication reconciliation between levels of care, patient and caregiver reports and information materials, and enhanced interoperability with other health systems and facilities. New functionalities of the system are also creating profound changes in workflow and patient engagement and optimization of the EHR continues via a process improvement strategy.

Shifting of Risk

More responsibility for the cost of care is being shifted from government and insurers to healthcare systems, providers, employers, and consumers. The stimulation of many healthcare models including accountable care organizations, patient-centered medical homes, bundled payments for disease states, and other advanced alternative payment models demonstrate different shared risk structures. Healthcare innovators acknowledge that there is risk in initiating new care models. Not all new models are hugely successful, especially early in implementation, and many require front-end investment in personnel and other resources.

New healthcare models such as ACOs assume greater financial risk for cost and health outcomes of the populations they cover. This wholesale transfer risks to others, both financial and outcome driven, produces profound effects. Is this ethical? What is the historical precedence? Approaches shifting more of the cost of employment-based health insurance visibly and directly into the household budgets of employees amount to rationing parts of the US healthcare system by price and ability to pay and also delegate an increasing amount of responsibility for cost to consumers [32].

References

1. ABIM Foundation, ACP–ASIM Foundation, and European Federation of Internal Medicine. Medical professionalism in the new millennium: a physician charter. Ann Intern Med. 2002;136(3):243–6.
2. Institute of Medicine (U.S.). Crossing the quality chasm: a new health system for the 21st century. Washington, DC: National Academy Press; 2001.
3. Fisher ES, Shortell SM, Savitz LA. Implementation science: a potential catalyst for delivery system reform. JAMA. 2016;315:339–40.

4. Zuckerman RB, Sheingold SH, Orav EJ, Ruhter J, Epstein AM. Readmissions, observation, and the hospital readmissions reduction program. N Engl J Med. 2016;374(16):1543–51.

5. Werner RM, Bradlow ET. Public reporting on hospital process improvements is linked to better patient outcomes. Health Aff (Millwood). 2010;29:1319–24.

6. Naylor M, Brooten D, Jones R, Lavizzo-Mourey R, Mezey M, Pauly M. Comprehensive discharge planning for the hospitalized elderly: a randomized clinical trial. Ann Intern Med. 1994;120:999–1006.

7. Coleman EA, Parry C, Chalmers S, Min SJ. The care transitions intervention: results of a randomized controlled trial. Arch Intern Med. 2006;166(17):1822–8.

8. Brewster AL, Cherlin EJ, Ndumele CD, et al. What works in readmissions reduction: how hospitals improve performance. Med Care. 2016;54(6):600–7.

9. Hernandez AF, Greiner MA, Fonarow GC, et al. Relationship between early physician follow-up and 30-day readmission among Medicare beneficiaries hospitalized for heart failure. JAMA. 2010;303:1716–22.

10. Ouslander JG, Bonner A, Herndon L, Shutes J. The interventions to reduce acute care transfers (INTERACT) quality improvement program: an overview for medical directors and primary care clinicians in long term care. J Am Med Dir Assoc. 2014;15:162–70.

11. Dharmarajan K, Wang Y, Lin Z, et al. Association of changing hospital readmission rates with mortality rates after hospital discharge. JAMA. 2017;318:270–8.

12. Americus Health Rankings Annual Report, 2017. https://www.americashealthrankings.org/learn/reports/2017-senior-report/executive-summary. Accessed 17 Nov 2017.

13. Wasfy JH, Zigler CW, Choriat C, Wang Y, Dominici F, Yeh RW. Readmission rate after passage of the hospital readmissions reduction program: a pre–post analysis. Ann Intern Med. 2017;166(5):324–31.

14. Kaiser Family Foundation. Aiming for fewer hospital U-turns: the Medicare hospital readmission reduction program. Washington, DC: Kaiser Family Foundation; 2017.

15. Joynt KE, Orav EJ, Zheng J, Jha AK. Public reporting of mortality rates for hospitalized Medicare patients and trends in mortality for reporting conditions. Ann Intern Med. 2016;165:153–60.

16. Krumholz HM, Normand SL, Wang Y. Trends in hospitalizations and outcomes for cardiovascular disease and stroke, 1999–2011. Circulation. 2014;130:966–75.

17. Joynt Maddox KE. Readmissions have declined, in mortality has not increased. The importance of evaluating the consequences. JAMA. 2017;318:243–4.

18. Desai NR, Ross JS, Kwon JY, et al. Association between hospital penalty status under the hospital readmission reduction program and readmission rates for target and nontarget conditions. JAMA. 2016;316:2647–56.

19. Centers for Medicare and Medicaid Services. Delivering better care at lower cost 9/16/14. https://www.cms.gov/Newsroom/MediaReleaseDatabase/Fact-sheets/2014-Fact-sheets-items/2014-09-16-2.html?DLPage=6&DLEntries=10&DLSort=0&DLSortDir=ascending. Accessed 17 Nov 2017.

20. Centers for Medicare and Medicaid Services. Bundled payments for care improvement (BPCI) initiative: General information. https://innovation.cms.gov/initiatives/bundled-payments. Accessed 28 Oct 2017.

21. Ryan AM, Krinsky S, Adler-Milstein J, Damberg C, Mauer KA, Hollingsworth JM. Association between hospitals engagement in value-based reforms and readmission reduction in the hospital readmissions reduction program. JAMA Intern Med. 2017;177:862–8.

22. Nyweide DJ, Lee W, Cuerdon TT, et al. Association of Pioneer accountable care organization vs traditional Medicare fee for service with spending, utilization, and patient experience. JAMA. 2015;313:2152–61.

23. Medicare Payment Advisory Commission. Data book: Beneficiaries dually eligible for Medicare and Medicaid — June 2017 MedPAC | MACPAC. http://www.medpac.gov/docs/default-source/data-book/jun17_databookentirereport_sec.pdf?sfvrsn=0. Accessed 17 Nov 2017.

24. Gurwitz JH, Bonner A, Berwick DM. Reducing excessive use of antipsychotic agents in nursing homes. JAMA. 2017;318:118–9.

25. Mendelson A, Kondo K, Damberg C, Low A, Motuapauka M, Freeman M, O'Neil M, Relevo R, Kansagara D. The effects of paper performance programs in health, health care use, and processes of care: a systematic review. Ann Intern Med. 2017;166:341–53.

26. Newhouse JP, McGuire TG. How successful is Medicare advantage? Milbank Q. 2014;92:351–94.

27. Casillas GM. What do we know about health care access and quality in Medicare Advantage versus the traditional Medicare program? Kaiser Family Foundation. 2014. http://www.kff.org/medicare/report/what-do-we-know-about-health-care-access-and-quality-in-medicare-advantage-versus-the-traditional-medicare-program/. Accessed 17 Nov 2017.

28. Chen LM, Epstein AM, Orav EJ, Filice CF, Samson LW, Joynt Maddox KE. Association of practice level social and medical risk with performance in the Medicare physician value-based payment modifier program. JAMA. 2017;318:453–61.

29. Joynt KE, De Lew N, Sheingold SH, Conway PH, Goodrich K, Epstein AM. Should Medicare value-based purchasing take social risk into account? N Engl J Med. 2017;376:510–3.

30. American Board of Internal Medicine Foundation. Choosing Wisely Campaign. www.choosingwisely.org. Accessed 17 Nov 2017.

31. Song Z, Chokski D. The role of private payers and payment reform. JAMA. 2015;313(1):25–6.

32. Reinhardt U. Healthcare price transparency and economics dairy. JAMA. 2014;312(16):1642–3.

Chapter 4
Value-Based Healthcare Purchasing

Abstract The US healthcare system is undergoing a value-based transformation. Value-based purchasing is a demand-side strategy to reward quality in healthcare delivery. The opportunities and challenges involved in value-based transformation are real and substantial. The scope of transformation of the US healthcare system includes all healthcare providers, healthcare systems, consumers, and healthcare educational institutions.

Core Measurements for Healthcare Systems

Value-based purchasing drives quality metrics which are publicly reported and serve as important levers for changes in healthcare delivery, promotes standardization, and reduces process variations. Measurement is essential to guide progress. Results and measures need to be reliable and consistent. We must measure what matters most, utilizing consistent core metrics to sharpen focus and improve performance. The Institute of Medicine (now called the National Academy of Medicine—NAM) report on vital signs forms a framework for 15 core measures of healthcare quality, value, and engagement, with focused goals for population health improvement [1] (Table 4.1).

© Springer International Publishing AG, part of
Springer Nature 2018
J. S. Powers, *Value Driven Healthcare and Geriatric Medicine*,
https://doi.org/10.1007/978-3-319-77057-4_4

TABLE 4.1 National academy of medicine: core measures of healthcare quality, value, and engagement

1. Life expectancy at birth
2. Self-reported health
3. Body mass index (BMI)
4. Addiction death rate
5. Teen pregnancy rate
6. High school graduation rate
7. Childhood immunization rate
8. Unmet care need reported
9. Hospital-acquired infection (HAI)
10. Preventable hospitalization rate
11. Patient–clinician communication
12. High spending relative to income
13. Per capita expenditures on health care
14. Health literacy rate
15. Social support

The challenge remains to define market benchmarks and measurable outcomes that providers will adopt. In primary care the benefits of continuity of care are generally acknowledged but we have yet to operationalize the measurement of continuity of care and its attributed costs to apply to downstream outcomes for primary care involvement. Similarly, we must learn to target resources, focusing on special-needs high-risk populations in order to make measurable progress on core values. New healthcare delivery models are needed which focus on standardization, transparency, competition, efficiency, and generation of quality outcomes (Table 4.2).

Interest continues to grow in pursuing the benefits of care delivery models designed to control costs and improve quality. Despite the large number of models being implemented,

TABLE 4.2 Healthcare
model evaluation

1. Standardization
2. Transparency
3. Competition
4. Efficiency
5. Quality outcomes

such as bundled disease episode payments and per-beneficiary payments to primary care groups in integrated healthcare organizations, the evidence for the effectiveness of these value-based models is mixed and limited. It becomes difficult to know which initiative should be scaled up and which models need further refinement or replaced in order to support a more efficient high-value healthcare system.

In order for pay-for-performance to be effective, the incentives must be the following: (1) large enough and temporally close to activity, (2) focus on a small number of high-value measures that will motivate clinicians to change behavior, and (3) the design must be simple enough for clinical and organizational leaders to obtain direct feedback to know how they are doing [2]. Physician acceptance and use of data determine how gaps in care and cost reduction are affected. It is challenging to obtain patient-specific data quickly enough to affect care outcomes in real time. Accurate data supported by real-time analytics technology as well as support for care coordination help get physicians engaged to achieve quality goals.

It is also important to develop appropriate use criteria based on best practices. For example, new guidelines for high-value care are being developed for more appropriate use of cardiac imaging techniques [3]. New ways of thinking about the costs and benefits of delivery models now include added emphasis on cost avoidance. No longer can we afford to make business decisions about program worth based on short-term economic considerations. We must also consider the costs to the system of *not* pursuing models that may have longer term downstream benefits but come with start-up resource requirements.

The critical source of cross subsidies from government has changed. Providers and healthcare organizations are realizing that pay for performance and quality outcome measurement are powerful forces altering previous roles of negotiating with private insurance which is no longer able to rely on cross subsidies from government programs. Interest in accountable care organizations (ACOs) has increased. ACOs curb costs and provide bonuses for hitting quality and cost benchmarks as well as global budget targets. The locus of risk for the cost of healthcare has shifted from government to insurers, healthcare organizations, providers, employers, and consumers. The movement in this direction is slow but continuous. There are powerful market forces involved in the value-based transformation of healthcare shaping a new paradigm where providers hold much more risk. In many metropolitan areas healthcare organizations have already assembled the components to develop integrated delivery systems. Many are now positioned to organize into ACOs equipped to bear financial risk. An integrated delivery system represents a collaborative effort. As risk is assumed, contributions to quality accrue across the healthcare continuum. For example, there is evidence of some significant reductions in post-acute spending without deterioration and quality of care related to participation in the Medicare Shared Savings Program (MSSP). In a 2012–2014 analysis of 114 accountable care organizations participating in MSSP, there was an overall reduction in post-acute spending driven by reductions in acute inpatient care, fewer discharges to facilities rather than home, and reduced length of SNF days. Also, participation in MSSP was not associated with significant changes in 30-day readmissions or use of highly rate–preferred skilled nursing facilities or mortality [4].

Competition and pricing are intimately related to the demographics of an aging population. Traditional Medicare (TM), Medicare Advantage (MA), commercial health insurance, and marketing practices greatly influence pricing and physician reimbursement. TM anchors prices, and serves as the comparison for MA which must achieve lower targets. MA currently covers less than half of the Medicare population, with room to grow. Healthcare systems operate with a portfolio of patients and insurers and consider all payer sources, commercial, TM, and MA, if the net revenue from the entire portfolio is attractive. Insurers subsidize the growth of their MA networks by paying higher rates for commercial patients. Commercial markup is particularly high for emergency room coverage. A reduction in the TM population may therefore drive cost increases unless regulations are in place to limit the amounts healthcare systems can bill for out-of-network commercial services [5, 6].

Guiding Principles for Quality Outcomes

CMS has defined better health care as improving the patient's experience of care within the NAM's six quality domains (Table 4.3). Keeping patients well so that they can do what they want to and increasing the overall health of populations should be the goals of a healthcare system. This includes addressing behavioral risk factors, and focuses on preventive care.

The American College of Physicians likewise, in its Charter on Medical Professionalism, emphasizes population health in its commitments linking professional care to the vision of improving the patient's and public's health [8] (Table 4.4).

Moreover, there is great disparity in healthcare outcomes that is not explained by cost. Geographic variation in healthcare costs in the Medicare fee-for-service population has fueled the perception of an inefficient US healthcare system

TABLE 4.3 National Academy of Medicine's six quality domains [7]	
	1. Safety
	2. Effectiveness
	3. Patient centeredness
	4. Timeliness
	5. Efficiency
	6. Equity

TABLE 4.4 American College of Physicians' Charter on Medical Professionalism

1. Commitment to improve the quality of care
2. Commitment to improve access to care
3. Commitment to just distribution of finite healthcare resources

which lacks transparency. Elucidating the causes of geographic variation and comparing the effects of new models of care on usual costs and processes of care are important priorities for comparative effectiveness research. A National Academy of Medicine report suggests that 73% of the variation is in post-acute care and 27% is attributed to inpatient care [9]. Healthcare transparency and accountability are increased with public accountability and reporting. Transparency can promote savings and standardization and encourage better quality.

All medical societies have now followed the lead of the American Board of Internal Medicine Foundation's Choosing Wisely Campaign [10] to promote high-value care principles. The American Board of Internal Medicine Foundation in collaboration with multiple other organizations is engaged in worldwide initiative to promote the practice of high-value care. The goals of the Choosing Wisely campaign are to improve healthcare outcomes by providing care with proven benefit in reducing costs by avoiding unnecessary and even harmful interventions. This includes the balancing of clinical benefit with costs or harms for a given intervention into a broad range of educational materials to address the needs of trainees, practicing physicians, and inpatients. High-value care recommendations include recommendations for diagnostic and management strategies for patients and specific clinical conditions and situations that balance clinical benefit with costs and harms with the goal of improving patient outcomes. There is some early evidence that there is more cost-conscious test ordering following the introduction of high-value healthcare recommendations [11]. Below are high-value care recommendations for primary care and geriatrics (Tables 4.5 and 4.6).

Table 4.5 High-value Care Recommendations—Primary Care examples [13]

1. Vaccination with herpes zoster vaccine is recommended for individuals aged 60 and older including patients with previous episode of zoster

2. Diagnostic testing for low back pain should be reserved for patients with severe progressive neurological deficits, patients in whom a serious underlying condition is suspected, or patients who do not have symptom improvement after 4–6 weeks

3. Routine antibiotic treatment of uncomplicated upper respiratory tract infections and acute bronchitis in a non-elderly immunocompetent patient is not indicated because of lack of efficacy and associated harms and costs

4. Hospital to primary provider communication at discharge, predischarge patient education, medication reconciliation, and a timely post-hospitalization follow-up are all necessary to improve patient safety during transitions of care

5. Palliative care medicine maximizes quality of life for patients with serious illnesses by meticulous symptom management and by aligning comprehensive care to meet the patient's goals as much as possible

A cross-sectional observation study derived from the National Ambulatory Medical Care Survey (2005–2013) and the National Hospital Ambulatory Medical Care Survey (2005–2011) indicated that 19–33% of primary care patients aged 18–64 received low-value medical services. The prevalence of low-value medical services provided was similar irrespective of insurance status, Medicaid, and lack of health insurance [12].

Risk Assessment

Traditional risk assessment or relative risk stratification (RRS) is derived from medical conditions, diagnoses, age, and sex [15]. This belies the known contribution of social and behavioral characteristics, or social determinants of health

TABLE 4.6 High-value Care Recommendations—Geriatrics examples [14]

1. Don't recommend percutaneous feeding tubes in patients with advanced dementia; instead offer oral assistance with feeding

2. Don't use antipsychotics as the first choice to treat behavioral and psychological symptoms of dementia

3. Avoid using medications other than metformin to achieve hemoglobin A_{1c} less than 7.5% in most older adults; moderate control is generally better

4. Don't use benzodiazepines or other sedatives in older adults as first choice for insomnia, agitation, or delirium

5. Don't use antimicrobials to treat bacteriuria in older adults unless specific urinary tract symptoms are present

6. Don't prescribe cholinesterase inhibitors for dementia without periodic assessment for perceived cognitive benefits and adverse gastrointestinal effects

7. Don't recommend screening for breast, colorectal, prostate, or lung cancer without considering life expectancy and risks of testing, over-diagnosis, and overtreatment

8. Avoid using appetite stimulants and high-calorie supplements for treatment of anorexia or cachexia in older adults; instead, optimize social supports, discontinue medications that may interfere with eating, provide appealing food and feeding assistance, and clarify patient goals and expectations

9. Don't prescribe a medication without conducting a drug regimen review

10. Don't use physical restraints to manage behavioral symptoms of hospitalized older adults with delirium

(SDH), to healthcare costs and outcomes. SDH includes serious mental health disorders, developmental disabilities, substance-use disorder, unstable housing, low income, unsafe neighborhoods, and substandard education [16]. A model that includes consideration of behavioral and social factors

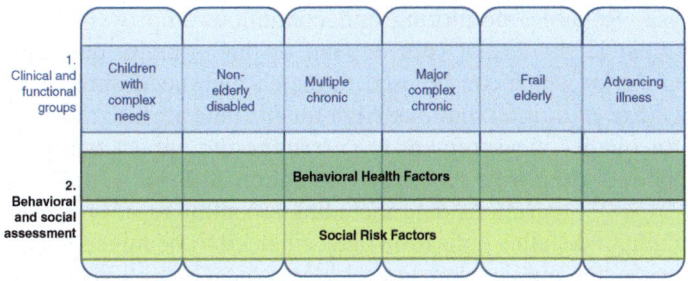

FIGURE 4.1 Risk assessment contributions to health outcomes [20]

related to health outcomes is depicted in Fig. 4.1. Allocation of payments to managed care organizations according to enrollees' social and medical risk may provide additional payments for socially vulnerable individuals that could fund support services, improve the match of payments to costs, and improve health equity [17, 18]. Indeed, social and behavioral determinants of health can even outperform disease-based factors in predicting outcomes, as shown in a study of a neighborhood disadvantage index (NDI) vs. the Pooled Cohort Equations Risk Model (PCERM) of the American College of Cardiology and the American Heart Association related to ASCVD 5-year event rates. PCERM performance worsened among patients living in resource-challenged neighborhoods and the NDI accounted for more than three times the amount of geographic variability in major ASCVD 5-year event rates [19]. The attribution of resources to special-needs populations may improve care for these groups, function as a strategy for cost containment, and appropriately value providers and services supporting high-risk, high-need populations.

Developing the Tools for Evaluation

Medicine needs the help of big data and informatics. The EHR positions us to ask pertinent questions to collaborate with data managers in the development and evaluation of integrated data measures for comparative effectiveness analysis. Reliable monitoring and continuous improvement of effective models of care depend on high-quality data and analytics which can be used to match high-need individuals with specific interventions. High-quality data are also required for quality measurement to determine the impact that care models are having on care coordination, utilization, and cost [21–24]. Operations data including a combination of enrollment and claims utilization data will need to be linked to risk modeling and development of hierarchical condition categories to define the functions and conditions related to episodes of care. We need to utilize big data to analyze outcomes, to develop new quality measures which identify and target high-risk populations, and to more appropriately evaluate programs and delivery systems. Risk value must also be determined in the context of the policy environment. Big data can help inform decision-making regarding the delivery quality and cost of care. Data resources must be harnessed to develop cost modeling based on risk scoring, informing risk-adjusted program evaluation, in order to target appropriate populations for screening, intervention services, and care coordination. Refinements in risk stratification modeling may ultimately feed back to shape healthcare policy (Table 4.7).

Quality Outcomes Assessment: Patient-Reported Outcomes

Standardization drives improvement; however risk assignment and adjustment for clinical and demographic healthcare settings are also important. Analysis of big data sets to identify longitudinal outcomes that enhance patient-centered goals is critical. Cross-sectional longitudinal data can help to inform systems-level performance outcomes. One example is the work of the International Consortium for Health Outcomes Measurement (ICHOM) which has produced a standard set of outcome measurements referable to older persons [25] (Fig. 4.2). However, patient-reported outcomes are also necessary to understand what matters most to

TABLE 4.7 Goals for development of data evaluation tools

1. Definition of episodes of care

   - Overlapping services and location of care

   - Tracking of care through different service utilization locations

   - Understanding of factors associated with different sites of care

2. Develop diagnosis-based and functional needs indices for

   - High-risk populations

   - Multi-morbidity

   - Prognosis-based care

3. Assess the distribution of diagnosis and functional needs indices across the population

4. Perform a longitudinal analysis to determine treatment effects

5. Develop program-based risk indices

6. Consider the time to benefit for screening procedures

7. Define the relationship of the provider to the patient

   - Episodic versus longitudinal care

   - Disease management versus continuity of care

   - Risk attribution

   - Cost attribution

8. Target the appropriate population and site of care

patients and to set performance priorities. The VA's Center for Health Equity Research and Promotion (formerly the PROMISE Center, now called the Veterans' Experience Center) Performance Reporting and Outcomes Measurement to Improve the Standard of care at End-of-life is another example of a program designed according to patient-centered goals of care. PROMISE's goals are (1) to identify and reduce

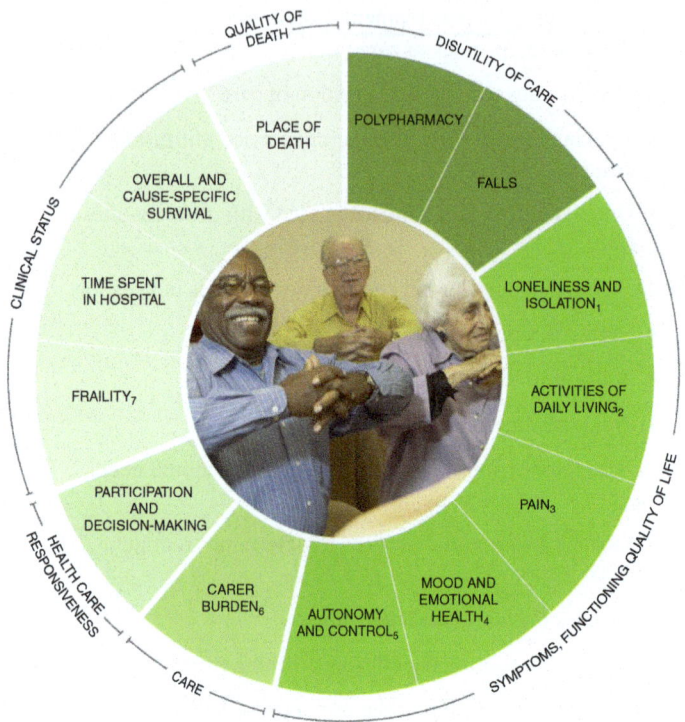

FIGURE 4.2 International Consortium for Health Outcomes Measurement (ICHOM), Standard Set for Older Persons

unwanted variation in the quality of end-of-life care throughout the VA, and (2) to define and disseminate processes of care ("best practices") that contribute to improved outcomes for veterans near the end of life and their families [26].

Example 4.1 Denver Health Whole Population Risk Stratification.

Denver Health received a CMS Innovation fund grant to develop a whole population risk stratification model. The goal was to improve the experience of care, improve the health of populations, improve provider engagement, and reduce per capita cost of healthcare. Denver Health's risk stratification approach used clinical risk groups (CRGs), a clinically based classification system originally developed by 3 M to measure the burden of illness in a population [27]. The stratification

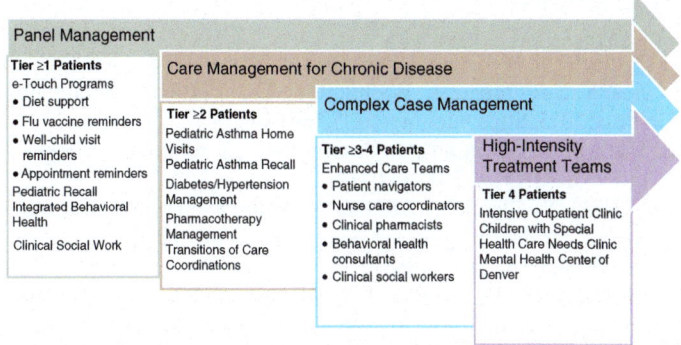

FIGURE 4.3 Denver Health Whole Population Risk Stratification [20]

used input from clinicians as well as data analysis to assign every CRG-classified patient to one of 14 years of increasing complexity and risk (Fig. 4.3).

For Tier 1 patients, the addition of e-touch text messaging to standard panel management techniques helped improve clinical outcomes including decreased no-show rates in higher immunization rates. Tier 2 patient management included late patient navigators, nurse care coordination, and some home visits. Tiers 3 and 4 patients (super-utilizers) received complex case management strategies with enhanced care teams as well as specialized intensive outpatient clinics addressing special needs utilizing a multidisciplinary approach to care. The intensive outpatient clinic was targeted to adults with multiple potentially avoidable inpatient admissions within the previous year and served as the patient's medical home. Over a 2-year period, only a small number of super-utilizers continuously met the super-utilizer criteria, although many went back and forth between meeting and not meeting those criteria. True cost savings were approximately 2% annually. In addition to having a significant clinical impact, the program produced a positive effect on family and pro-vider satisfaction and demonstrates the power of a population-based stratification system that is sustainable based on financial performance [20].

References

1. Institute of Medicine. Vital signs: core metrics for health and health care progress. Washington, DC: National Academies Press; 2015. https://doi.org/10.17226/19402.
2. Jha AK. Value-based purchasing: time for rebound or time to move on? JAMA. 2017;317:1107–8.
3. Doukky R, Diemer G, Medina A, et al. Promoting appropriate use of cardiac imaging: no longer an academic exercise. Ann Intern Med. 2017;166:438–40.
4. McWilliams JM, Gilstrap LG, Stevenson DG, et al. Changes in post-acute care and the Medicare shared savings program. JAMA Intern Med. 2017;177:518–26.
5. Trish E, Ginsburg P, Gascue L, Geoffrey J. Physician reimbursement in Medicare advantage compared with traditional Medicare and commercial health insurance. JAMA Int Med. 2017;177:1287–95.
6. Robinson JC. Medicare advantage reimbursement to physicians. JAMA Int Med. 2017;177:1295–6.
7. The National Academies of Science, Engineering, and Medicine. Crossing the quality chasm: a new health system for the 21st Century. http://nationalacademies.org/hmd/reports/2001/crossing-the-quality-chasm-a-new-health-system-for-the-21st-century.aspx. Accessed 17 Nov 2017.
8. ABIM Foundation. ACP, European Federation of Internal Medicine. Medical professionalism in the new millennium: a physician charter. Ann Intern Med. 2002;136:243–6.
9. Institute of Medicine. Interim report of the committee on geographic variation in health care spending and promotion of high value care: preliminary committee observations. http://books.nap.edu/openbook.php?record_id=18308. Accessed 17 Nov 2017.
10. Johnson PT, Pahwa AK, Feldman LS, Ziegelstein RC, Hellmann DB. Advancing high-value healthcare: a new AJM column dedicated to cost-conscious care quality improvement. Am J Med. 2017;130:619–20.
11. American Board of Internal Medicine Foundation. Choosing Wisely Campaign. www.choosingwisely.org. Accessed 17 Nov 2017.
12. Barnett ML, Linder JA, Ckark CR, Sommers BD. Low value medical services in the safety net population. JAMA Intern Med. 2017;177:829–37.

13. American College of Physicians medical knowledge self-assessment program, 17, American College of Physicians, c 2015, Philadelphia.
14. American Geriatrics Society. Choosing wisely campaign. 2015. http://www.choosingwisely.org/societies/american-geriatrics-society/. Accessed 17 Nov 2017.
15. Kautter J, Pope CG, Ingber M, et al. The HHS-HCC risk adjustment model for individual and small group markets under the affordable care act. Medicare Medicaid Res Rev. 2014;4:E1–E11.
16. The Centers for Disease Control. Social determinants of health. https://www.cdc.gov/socialdeterminants/. Accessed 7 Oct 2017.
17. Ash A, Mick EO, Ellis RP, Kiefe C, Allison JJ, Clark M. Social determinants of health and managed care payment formulas. JAMA Intern Med. 2017;177:1424–30.
18. Joynt Maddox K. Social and behavioral determinants of spending. JAMA Intern Med. 2017;177:1431–2.
19. Dalton JE, Perzynski AT, Zidar DA, Rothberg MB, Coulton CJ, Milnovich AT, Einstadter D, Karichu JK, Dawson NV. Accuracy of cardiovascular risk prediction varies by neighborhood socioeconomic position: a retrospective cohort study. Ann Int Med. 2017;167:456–64.
20. National Academy of Medicine. Effective care for high need patients: opportunities for improving outcomes, value, and health. https://nam.edu/initiatives/clinician resilience-and-well-being/effective-care-for-high-need-patients/. Accessed 17 Nov 2017.
21. Bates DW, Saria S, Ohno-Machado L, Shah A, Escobar G. Big data in health care: using analytics to identify and manage high-risk and high-cost patients. Health Aff. 2014;33(7):11231131.
22. Bradley EH, Canavan M, Rogan E, Talbert-Slagle K, Ndumele C, Taylor L, Curry LA. Variation in health outcomes: the role of spending on social services, public health, and health care, 2000-09. Health Aff. 2016;35(5):760–8.
23. Dale SB, Ghosh A, Peikes DN, Day TJ, Yoon FB, Taylor EF, Swankoski K, O'Malley AS, Conway PH, Rajkumar R, Press MJ, Sessums L, Brown R. Two-year costs and quality in the comprehensive primary care initiative. N Engl J Med. 2016;374(24):2345–56.
24. Rajkumar R, Press MJ, Conway PH. The CMS innovation center-a five-year self-assessment. N Engl J Med. 2015;372(21):1981–3.
25. http://www.ichom.org/medical-conditions/older-person/. Accessed 17 Nov 2017.

26. https://www.cherp.research.va.gov/PROMISE/index.asp. Accessed 17 Nov 2017.
27. Hughes JS, Averill RF, Eisenhandler J, Goldfield NI, Muldoon J, Neff JM, Gay JC. Clinical risk groups (CRGs): a classification system for risk-adjusted capitation-based payment and health care management. Med Care. 2004;42:81–90.

Chapter 5
New Models of Healthcare Delivery

Abstract The United States is in the midst of a bold experiment. The transformation of the healthcare system has stimulated numerous alternative payment models and many new models of care. There is an array of new healthcare delivery models with varying scope and magnitude of risk for providers. Quality metrics are the outcome measures by which these new models are evaluated.

Effective Care

The Agency for Healthcare Research and Quality (AHRQ) reports that 50% of healthcare costs occur among 5% of the US population (2002) [1]. In the United States approximately 1% of patients account for more than 20% of all healthcare expenditures. Program targeting for added services for high-risk populations, focusing services to needs, makes sense (Fig. 5.1).

High-need adults with three or more chronic conditions and functional limitations average over $21,000 yearly in healthcare and prescription costs. This is more than four times the average for all US adults, and almost three times more than adults with three or more chronic conditions but without functional limitations (Fig. 5.2) [4].

© Springer International Publishing AG, part of   65
Springer Nature 2018
J. S. Powers, *Value Driven Healthcare and Geriatric Medicine*,
https://doi.org/10.1007/978-3-319-77057-4_5

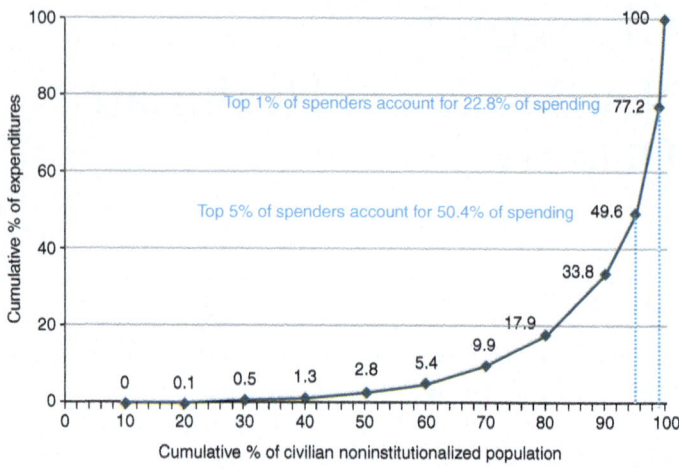

FIGURE 5.1 Distribution of personal healthcare spending in the US Civilian Noninstitutionalized population, 2014 [2, 3]

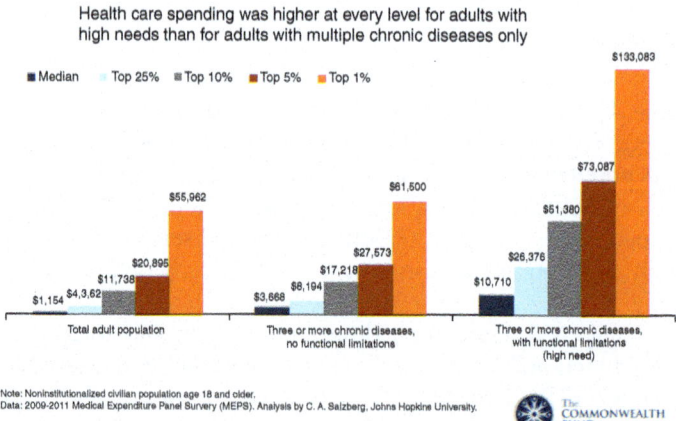

FIGURE 5.2 High-need adults had higher spending on health care than did those with three or more chronic conditions without functional limitations. *Reproduced with permission of the Commonwealth Fund*

The high-need population is characterized by three criteria: total healthcare costs, intensity of care utilization for a given period of time, and having functional self-care limitations [2]. In addition to attending to clinical needs, the high-need population also requires addressing behavioral, functional, and social needs with enhanced provision of social and community support services [5].

The Scope of Change

Medicare is moving away from traditional fee-for-service to alternative payment models (APMs) intended to improve quality and reduce costs. However, these models are still being implemented and tested. All physicians and healthcare systems are reacting to the demise of fee-for-service and adapting to new models of care. The stakes are high; on the other hand, payment and policy inform the adoption and dissemination of new models of care. This is an exciting opportunity to infuse and mainstream geriatric healthcare models and principles into healthcare systems.

The delivery transformation stimulated by value-based purchasing is forcing healthcare systems to evaluate the effects of different components of service along the continuum of care. These considerations include cost as well as risk. Many health systems however remain hospital centric with limited sharing of resources with other components along the continuum of care. It is encouraging however that many innovative delivery models are emerging, stimulated by the CMS Innovation Center, the Veterans Administration, and other healthcare systems intent on improving outcomes and fueled by value-based purchasing. Value-based healthcare transformation is also exerting a tremendous amount of leverage on providers in the form of conditions of participation. Commercial payer contracts are also increasingly influenced by value-based reimbursement models.

Delivery Models

Care models that have been successful in addressing the care of high-need patients foster effectiveness across three domains: (1) health and well-being, (2) care utilization, and (3) costs. Successful models of care can be graded across four dimensions: (1) the service setting, (2) care attributes, (3) delivery features, and (4) organizational culture. Service setting includes a focus on managing high-need and frequent utilizers, including enhanced primary care, transitional care, and integrated care. Care attributes include elements of assessment, targeting, planning, communication and coordination of care, patient and caregiver training, and outreach and patient monitoring. Organizational culture contributing to the success of care models includes engagement of leadership across levels of care, adapting the model to local contexts, strong team relationships, and continuous assessment utilizing multiple data sources [7].

Single disease management programs were initially based on limited observations. These programs fell out of favor when more rigorous evaluations failed to confirm their cost savings. One notable exception however was the Medicare Diabetes Prevention Program.

Bundled Payments for Care Improvement (BPCI) is a voluntary program phased in between 2013 and 2015 in which some 1400 organizations are currently participating. Participants can select up to 48 different clinical episodes and the choice determines the bundled payments. The parent organization managing the bundled payment is responsible for determining specific reimbursement amounts for all facilities and providers. Payments are made from the funds received in the bundled payment, which is made retrospectively. The amount of payment is based on historical payments, less a discount. If the organization is below target, it will receive a share of the cost savings. The model entails risk bearing if total cost for the episode exceeds the target price, but participating organizations also share some portion of the cost savings with CMS. One of the questions surrounding bundled payments is whether the effort to align financial incentives between physicians and hospitals could contribute to increases in volume or shifts in case mix towards healthier and more profitable patients. Bundled payments make it easier to engage specialists and smaller hospital physician practices, encouraging care coordination across clinical sites of care. This may help reduce avoidable post-acute institutional-based care. Importantly however, bundled payments leave the incentive to increase volume solidly in place.

Bundled payment models are being expanded to include additional conditions, particularly surgical procedures. These include joint replacement, valve replacement, CABG, acute myocardial infarction, and stroke bundles. These models are protocol driven with evidence-based best practices built into each component.

There is limited information on BCPI outcomes and quality measures. In the first 21 months of the total joint replacement (TJR) bundled care initiative (includes all related care services including a 90-day post-discharge visit), Medicare payments declined more for lower extremity joint replacement episodes provided in BCPI participating hospitals than for those provided in comparison hospitals without any significant change in quality outcomes [6]. Almost all the reduction in spending was from reduced use of institutional post-acute care. There is also a trend towards healthier patients in the BPCI hospitals than in the comparison group, although population-based rates of total joint replacement vary widely across the US Hospital Referral Regions.

The BPCI payment model may encourage hospitals to improve transitions and post-discharge monitoring since variations in post-acute spending are major drivers of regional differences in Medicare spending. Episode-based payments may reduce the use of post-acute services that are of low value or unnecessary. The risk of future adverse events dictates the optimal treatment course, and claims data may not adequately assess this risk. For instance, traumatic hip fractures are currently included in the joint replacement bundle. CMS may encounter challenges in determiningwhether more expensive treatments are being used appropriately or avoided. The 90-day current episode-based payment following the index hospitalization may also create incentives to avoid excessive or expensive care that improves long-term outcomes.

For the Oncology Care Model (OCM) and the Comprehensive Care for Joint Replacement Model (CJR), hospitals bear financial risk or receive rewards based on episode-level spending and quality. This is similar to the two-sided risk, population-based global payment contracts for accountable care organizations (ACOs). If spending is below budget there is a reward and a penalty if spending exceeds the budget. Incentives for the 90-day episodes are phased in over 5 years to protect beneficiaries from incentives for under-utilization of care. Hospitals may keep no more than 5% of the episode-based payments in the first 2 years and no more than 10%, 20%, and 20%, respectively, in the last 3 years of the contract. In contrast to planned chemotherapy and elective joint replacement surgery, events in the acute myocardial infarction bundle are unanticipated. Outcomes after an acute MI are heavily influenced by cardiac rehabilitation, but the adoption of cardiac rehabilitation is highly variable among BPCI participants.

In the BPCI model, hospital evaluations are shifted from hospital to regional-based benchmarks which produce some incentives to reduce variation, but could also weaken the link between hospitals' absolute improvement in performance. Hospitals resourced with higher cost capabilities may spend more but remain below their quality benchmark. Indeed hospitals with higher operating margins are associated with lower rates of BPCI dropout [7]. Stratifying benchmarks by hospital resources or providing greater rewards for participation could help address these concerns.

ACOs are provided a prospective payment to manage a local population of Medicare patients selected by CMS. Global budgeting is not a new idea. The health maintenance organizations (HMOs) of the 1990s developed into preferred provider organizations (PPOs), which were characterized by selection of favorable patient populations. But ACOs have populations assigned by CMS to equitably distribute risk within patient populations. There is a gradual phase-in of risk over a 3-year period with an initial shared savings and then adding of downside risk and a greater potential for profits. As of 2016 Leavitt Partners, in partnership with the Accountable Care Learning Collaborative, estimated that there are 838 ACOs nationwide covering 28.3 million lives [8]. Early information suggests that ACOs are indeed driving value-based care, increasing overall quality reporting scores from 70 to 84% [9].

Accountable care organizations create consolidation of medical services. There are some concerns about the harms of consolidation, about the amount of risk bearing needed to produce changes in behavior, and how to manage shared resources and potential financial conflicts between different health system components in ACOs. Hospitals may retain savings from inpatient-related bundles for patients attributed to the entire ACO. Some ACOs have global budgets with substantial downside risk, and others such as Medicare Shared Savings Plans (MSSP) are shared savings programs where participating organizations receive bonus payments for meeting budget goals, but bear no downside risk. The amount of financial risk bearing necessary to achieve behavior change is an important area of inquiry and very little is known about this [10].

Care Models for High-Need Patients

The National Academy of Medicine report on improving care for high-need patients offers 14 specific evidence-based care models that payers can support and which systems can implement [2]. These successful care models highlight many of the attributes delivery features and operational practices designed to improve care for high-need patients including interdisciplinary primary care: guided care, the Program for All-inclusive Care for the Elderly—PACE [11–13]; care and case management: Massachusetts General Physicians Organization

Integrated Care Management Program [13]; transitional care: Naylor Transitional Care Model [15–17]; and programs with strong integration of medical, social, and behavioral services: Improving Mood: Promoting Access to Collaborative Treatment—IMPACT [18–21]. A crosswalk of these programs and the high-need segments of the population served is depicted in Fig. 5.3. Successful programs applying to adults are described in detail below.

Geriatrics is unique among specialties in having developed a large array of wide-ranging, successful programs that improve the quality of life of older persons who consume so many healthcare resources. These programs contribute greatly to new models of healthcare delivery.

Program \ Segment	Children w/ complex needs	Non-elderly disabled	Multiple chronic	Major complex chronic	Frail elderly	Advancing illness
Care management plus				*		*
Commonwealth care alliance						
Complex care program at Children's National Health system						
GRACE				*		
Guided care						
Health quality partners						
Health services for children with special needs	*					
Hospital at home						
H-PACT		*				
IMPACT			*		*	
Massachusetts general physicians organization care management program						
MIND at home					*	
Naylor transitional care model (Penn)						
PACE						

FIGURE 5.3 Successful care models for high-need patients [2]

The Massachusetts General Physicians Organization Integrated Care Management Program utilizes an interdisciplinary care management team targeting high-need patients for primary care practices. It has been found to improve coordination and reduce cost of care compared to traditional fee-for-service care [22].

Geriatric Resources for Assessing Care for Elders (GRACE) team care is a recent cost-effective team... care model that improves the health of frail older adults by working with patients in their homes and communities to manage health problems, track changing care needs, and leverage social services. In the GRACE model, interdisciplinary teams guided by care protocols improve outcomes. Increases in preventive and chronic care are offset by reduced acute care costs [23].

The Program for All-inclusive Care for Elderly (PACE) provides integrated acute medical care and long-term care services to frail seniors. PACE provides a community-based alternative to nursing home care when nursing home placement seems necessary. PACE uses blended Medicare and Medicaid financing to provide care, and reduces mortality and improves function [24]. Present since the 1970s, the costs of PACE home-based long-term care are offset by avoidance of nursing home costs. There are 233 PACE programs operating in 31 states and serving about 40,000 nursing home-eligible individuals [25].

Transitions of care programs for home care following hospitalization utilizing advance-practice nurse-directed discharge planning and follow-up protocols have shown promise in reducing early repeat hospitalizations [26]. Similarly, the Coleman Care Transitions Program, a patient-centered, self-management program coordinated by a health coach, has also reduced repeat hospitalizations [27]. Some 25% of post-acute care patients are readmitted to hospital within 30 days [28]. INTERACT is a nursing home quality improvement intervention providing tools and strategies to assist nursing home staff in the early identification, assessment, and communication and decision-making regarding changes in resident status.

TABLE 5.1 INTERACT strategies to reduce post-acute care hospital readmissions

Prevent conditions from becoming emergent requiring transfer
Manage some conditions with guidelines
Improve communication between all healthcare providers
Improve advance directive care planning
Integrate prevention of hospital readmission into quality assessment and performance improvement (QAPI) activities in the long-term care facility

INTERACT has been shown to reduce readmissions from post-acute care by 17–24% depending on the degree of facility engagement [29]. Table 5.1 lists the INTERACT strategies to reduce post-acute care hospital readmissions, which have also been applied to assisted-living facilities and home care. The improved communication and handoffs between hospital and nursing home appears to prevent avoidable rehospitalizations. There is potential to reduce the percentage of hospital readmissions from post-acute care institutions which are rated as potentially avoidable. However, the ratings and factors underlying avoidability differ between hospital and nursing home staff, supporting the need for joint accountability and collaboration for future readmission reduction efforts between hospitals and their post-acute care partners [30].

Improving Mood: Promoting Access to Collaborative Treatment—IMPACT targets older adults with depression and includes collaborative care in a care manager. The primary care physician works with a consulting psychiatrist and care manager to develop and implement a treatment plan which may include medication and counseling. This program helps identify depression among primary care patients, and has been effective in reducing depressive symptoms and total cost of health care among intervention patients as compared to a control group [20, 21].

The MIND at Home Program targets elderly patients with memory disorders. This home-based program links individuals with dementia and their caregivers to community-based agencies and healthcare providers as well as community resources. An interdisciplinary team delivers individualized care planning for patients and caregivers and monitors outcomes. Patients in the MIND at Home Program were able to stay in their homes average of 288 extra days over a 2-year follow-up and caregivers received more support compared with a control group receiving no special care [31–34].

Nurses Improving the Care of Health System Elders (NICHE) is dedicated to the principle that all older adults be given sensitive and exemplary care. The program began in 1981 and is now operating in 450 US hospitals. NICHE helps participating hospitals build nursing leadership capabilities to enact system-level changes targeting the unique needs of older adults and put evidence-based knowledge into practice. NICHE tools exert important influences over care provided to older adult patients by increasing the organizational support for geriatric nursing [35].

The Hospital at Home is designed to care for defined illnesses such as urinary tract infections, pneumonia, COPD exacerbation, and cellulitis in order to avoid hospitalization. Patients receive daily visits from a nurse with physician support available by phone. The team also includes a nurse practitioner, social worker, pharmacist, and dietitian. A Hospital at Home (admission avoidance) program seeks to provide hospital-level care for selected patients in the patient's home. Operating as an enhanced interdisciplinary team home care program, this model shows promise of achieving hospital quality standards with shorter lengths of stay for some condition such as pneumonia and urinary tract infection. There are also suggestions of reduced complications in addition to increased family and patient satisfaction [36].

Avoiding readmission within 30 days is a huge concern for hospitals and healthcare systems. There are many hospital-initiated post-discharge interventions (HiPDI), including phone calls to discharge patients within 48 h, and outpatient visits scheduled within 2 weeks of hospital discharge, home health visits, as well as enhanced home care such as Home-

Based Primary Care (HBPC), the VA's interdisciplinary team-based home care program. The Independence at Home Medicare demonstration projects bring primary care to Medicare patients, integrating care focusing on comorbidities and caregiver support. A meta-analysis of this demonstration program suggests that it also contributes to reduced 30-day readmission rates [37].

Acute Care for Elderly (ACE) Units provide interdisciplinary care, comprehensive review, and an environment of care conducive to early rehabilitation and patient-centered care, improving function and reducing iatrogenic and hospital-acquired conditions. A review of ACE Unit outcomes indicated that medical review, early rehabilitation, and patient-centered care with implementation of standardized and individualized function-focused interventions appeared to be optimal for overall outcome achievement compared to more limited discharge planning efforts [38]. These geriatric laboratories present since the 1970s, however, remain few in number nationally.

It is important to note that many of these healthcare innovations all come with variable degrees of risk tied to reimbursement strategies (Table 5.2).

Innovations in care delivery and care coordination for transitions of care include hospital-based nurse care managers meeting the patient prior to discharge, integration of care plans with the hospital team, and treating patients by protocol-driven post-discharge phone contact. Another model of post-discharge care for noncritical post-op patients includes co-management by primary care and surgery. This model also provides an individualized enhanced home health program with aggressive rehabilitation-oriented care to decrease length of stay in hospital.

TABLE 5.2 Comparativehealthcare delivery models (partial listing of models)

Model	Scope	Risk	Risk magnitude	Quality metrics
Global budget for Dual eligibles	Comprehensive care	Full		Population health
ACOs	Hospital referral area	Partial and full		Network goals
MSSP	Hospital referral area	Partial		Network goals
PACE	Network	Full		Network goals
PCMH	Limited	Partial		Primary care quality indicators
Bundled payment	Disease state	Full		Specialty care quality indicators
PPOs	Practices	Partial		Primary care and specialty quality indicators

Dual Eligibles low income, eligible for Medicaid and Medicare, *ACO* Accountable Care Organization, *MSSP* Medicare Shared Savings Plan, *PACE* Program for All-Inclusive Care of the Elderly, *PCMH* Patient Centered Medical Home, *PPO* Preferred Provider Organization

Assessing home health patients using a resident assessment for home care revealed multiple modifiable risk factors for unplanned hospitalization. Systematic assessment by multidisciplinary team at the beginning of service and targeting modifiable risk factors could reduce the risk of unplanned hospitalizations [39]. Care coordination for home care patients utilizing shift reports through a shared electronic health record (EHR) informs communication within the interdisciplinary team primary care providers [40].

CMS's Advancing Excellent in Nursing Home Care, now called the National Nursing Home Quality Improvement Campaign, is utilizing an educational approach to encourage facilities to adapt the nine goals of person-centered long-term care in their Quality Assessment and Performance Improvement (QAPI) programs [41]. The goals of person-centered long-term care are listed in Table 5.3.

Many other new care models are too new to have robust results. The patient-centered medical home provides increased care between visits, is nurse managed, and is associated with as many as 20% fewer required return outpatient visits, expanding the opportunity for new patients [42]. This model however requires initial investment of approximately 2.5 personnel per full-time practicing clinician and uptake has historically been slow under fee-for-service models. Telehealth or clinic-based video telehealth (CVT) visits for mental health, dementia, palliative care, and nursing home care patients has been very effective for goals of care discussion, symptom management, and caregiver support and provides more immediate consultation services for patients including a distance from major medical centers [43].

Emergency rooms are experiencing increased utilization. From 2003 to 2009 there was a 17% increase in admissions

TABLE 5.3 CMS nine goals of person-centered long-term care

Consistent assignment strengthens the relationship between caregivers, residents, and family
Hospitalization: Residents are often transferred to the hospital when they have an acute change in condition. Some conditions can be managed safely without transfer
Person-centered: Here promotes choices, purpose, and meaning in daily life
Staff stability: Most residents are comfortable with caregivers they know
Infections: Nursing homes are the most common place for *C. difficile* and other serious infections
Medications: Potentially inappropriate medications (PIMS) can compromise resident well-being
Mobility: Enhancing and maintaining mobility maintain physical and psychological well-being
Pain: Inadequate pain management can affect activity and quality of life
Pressure ulcers can be painful and dangerous to residents

from emergency room and a corresponding 10% decrease in admissions from office practices, suggesting that office-based physicians are increasingly relying on emergency departments to evaluate complex patients with potentially serious problems [44]. Another key driver of unnecessary emergency room use is lack of access to primary care. Some potential ways to improve care transitions in the emergency department to reduce return to the emergency department include case management, reducing potentially unnecessary medications [45], and improved coordination with primary care and specialty practices.

Healthcare hotspotting is a data-driven process developed by the Camden Coalition of healthcare providers for the timely identification of outlier patterns in a defined region of the healthcare system. Hotspotting utilizes claims data to guide targeted intervention and follow-up to better address patient needs, improve care quality, and reduce cost. Hotspotting can help reveal both a community's healthcare problems and their solutions and identify heavy utilizers to focus on this population [46].

Elements of the patient-centered medical home can be infused into healthcare systems with benefits to patients as well as the healthcare system. Proactive home visits utilizing paramedics provide level I patient assessments to frail and homebound elderly, engaging community supports and providing critical information to primary care providers. Paramedics trained in geriatric principles have been able to provide assessments of general health, frailty, social, cognitive, and functional abilities and share this information with primary care providers in order to develop care plans, obtain appropriate referrals, and introduce interventions. The Toronto Common Health Evaluation Completed Using Paramedicine Services (CHECUPS) that has permitted the development of partnerships with community providers has been found to benefit elderly individuals who are frequent utilizers of the healthcare system and to correct modifiable issues [47] and has shown a 47% reduction in 911 calls within a 6-month period [48]. Some models are also operating in the United States, termed mobile integrated healthcare and community paramedicine (EMS-MIH-CP), an emerging healthcare trend that is improving the lives of patients and transforming the role of the nation's emergency medical services, paramedics, and emergency medical technicians (EMTs).

Identifying the populations at risk, their true cost of care, and the value added for focused care management programs remain a challenge. We need to evolve the healthcare system to explore and value the interactive effects of complementary programs. We desperately need risk assessment models to effectively target interventions and innovative models of care for high-risk populations.

References

1. Agency for Healthcare Research and Quality. 2006. The high concentration of US healthcare expenditures. Pub 06–0060. https://meps.ahrq.gov/data_files/publications/st455/stat455.pdf. Accessed 17 Nov 2017.
2. National Academy of Medicine. Effective care for high need patients: opportunities for improving outcomes, value, and health. Chapters 2, 3. https://nam.edu/initiatives/clinician-resilience-and-well-being/effective-care-for-high-need-patients/. Accessed 17 Nov 2017.
3. Dzau VJ, McClellan MB, McGinnis J, et al. Vital directions for health and health care: priorities from a national academy of medicine initiative. JAMA. 2017;317(14):1461–70.
4. Hayes, S. L., C. A. Salzberg, D. McCarthy, D. C. Radley, M. K. Abrams, T. Shah, and G. F. Anderson. 2016. High-need, high-cost patients: who are they and how do they use health care? New York: The Commonwealth Fund. http://www.commonwealthfund.org/publications/issue-briefs/2016/dec/high-need-patients-experience-health-care. Accessed 17 Nov 2017.
5. Blumenthal D, Anderson G, Burke S, Fulmer T, Jha AK, and Long P. 2016. Tailoring complex-care management, coordination, and integration for high-need, high-cost patients: a vital direction for health and health care. In Discussion paper, edited by National Academy of Medicine. Washington, DC.
6. Dummit LA, Kahvecioglu D, Marrufo G, Rajkumar R, Marchall J, Tan E, Press MJ, Flood S, Muldoon L, Gu Q, Hassol A, Dott DM, Bassano A, Conway PH. Association between hospital participation in a Medicare bundled payments initiative and payment and quality outcomes for lower extremity joint replacement episodes. JAMA. 2016;316(12):1267–78.
7. Joynt-Maddox KE, Orav EJ, Zheng J, Epstein AM. Participation and dropout in the bundled payments for care improvement initiative. JAMA. 2018;319:191–3.
8. http://healthaffairs.org/blog/2016/04/21/accountable-care-organizations-in-2016-private-and-public-sector-growth-and-dispersion/. Accessed 17 Nov 2017.

9. Centers for Medicare and Medicaid Services. Delivering Better Care at Lower Cost 9/16/14. https://www.cms.gov/Newsroom/MediaReleaseDatabase/Fact-sheets/2014-Fact-sheets-items/2014-09-16-2.html?DLPage=6&DLEntries=10&DLSort=0&DLSortDir=ascending. Accessed 17 Nov 2017.

10. Colla CH, Fisher ES. Moving forward with accountable care organizations: some answers, more questions. JAMA Intern Med. 2017;177:527–8.

11. Boult C, Wieland GD. Comprehensive primary care for older patients with multiple chronic conditions: "nobody rushes you through.". JAMA. 2010;304:1936–43.

12. Hirth V, Baskins J, Dever-Bumba M. Program of all-inclusive care (PACE): past, present, and future. J Am Med Dir Assoc. 2009;10:155–60.

13. Lynch M, Hernandez M, Estes C. PACE: has it changed the chronic care paradigm? Soc Work Public Health. 2008;23:3–24.

14. Massachusetts general physicians organization integrated care management program. http://www.massgeneral.org/integrated-care-management/. Accessed 17 Nov 2017.

15. Bradway CR, Trotta MB, Bixby E, McPartland MC, Wollman H, Kapustka K, McCauley K, Naylor MD. A qualitative analysis of an advanced practice nurse-directed transitional care model intervention. Gerontologist. 2012;52:394–407.

16. Hirschman KB, Shaid E, McCauley K, Pauly MV, Naylor MD. Continuity of care: the transitional care model. Online J Issues Nurs. 2015;20:1.

17. Naylor MD. A decade of transitional care research with vulnerable elders. J Cardiovasc Nurs. 2000;14:1–14. quiz 88-19.

18. Callahan CM, Kroenke K, Counsell SR, Hendrie HC, Perkins AJ, Katon W, Noel PH, Harpole L, Hunkeler EM, Unutzer J. Treatment of depression improves physical functioning in older adults. J Am Geriatr Soc. 2005;53:367–73.

19. Lin EH, Katon W, Von Korff M, Tang L, Williams JW, Kroenke K, Hunkeler E, Harpole L, Hegel M, Arean P, Hoffing M, Della Penna R, Langston C, Unutzer J. Effect of improving depression care on pain and functional outcomes among older adults with arthritis: a randomized controlled trial. JAMA. 2003;290:2428–9.

20. Unutzer J, Katon W, Callahan CM, Williams JW, Hunkeler E, Harpole L, Hoffing M, Della Penna RD, Noel PH, Lin EH, Arean PA, Hegel MT, Tang L, Belin TR, Oishi S, Langston C. Collaborative care management of late-life depression in

the primary care setting: a randomized controlled trial. JAMA. 2002;288:2836–45.

21. Unutzer J, Katon WJ, Fan MY, Schoenbaum MC, Lin EC, Della Penna RD, Powers D. Long-term cost effects of collaborative care for late-life depression. Am J Manag Care. 2008;14:95–100.

22. Van Leeuwen Williams E, Unutzer J, Lee S, Noel PH. Collaborative depression care for the old-old: findings from the impact trial. Am J Geriatr Psychiatr. 2009;17:1040–9.

23. Counsell SR, Callahan CM, Tu W, Stump TE, Arling GW. Cost analysis of the geriatric resources for assessment and care of elders care management intervention. J Am Geriatr Soc. 2009;57:1420–6.

24. National PACE Association. PACE facts and trends. http://www.npaonline.org/policy-and-advocacy/pace-facts-and-trends-0. Accessed 17 Nov 2017.

25. Mason DJ. Long–term care: investigating in models at work. JAMA. 2017;318:1529–30.

26. Naylor MD, Brooten DA, Campbell RL, Maislin G, McCauley KM, Schwartz JS. Transitional care of older adults hospitalized with heart failure: a randomized, controlled trial. J Am Geriatr Soc. 2004;52:675–84.

27. Coleman EA, Smith JD, Frank JC, Min S, Parry C, Kramer AM. Preparing patients and caregivers to participate in care delivered across settings: the care transitions intervention. J Am Geriatr Soc. 2004;42:1817–25.

28. Mor V, Intrator O, Ferg Z, Grabowski DC. The revolving door of hospitalization from skilled nursing facilities. Health Aff. 2010;29:57–64.

29. Ouslander J, Lamb G, Tappan R, et al. Interventions to reduce hospitalizations from nursing homes: evaluation of the INTERACT II collaborative quality improvement project. J Am Geriatr Soc. 2011;59:745–53.

30. Vasilevskis EE, Ouslander JG, Mixon AS, Bell SP, Jacobsen JM, Saraf AA, Markley D, Sponsler KC, Shutes J, Long EA, Kripalani S, Simmons SF, Schnelle JF. Potentially avoidable readmissions of patients discharged to post-acute care: perspectives of hospital and skilled nursing facility staff. J Am Ger Soc. 2017;65:269–76.

31. Black BS, Johnston D, Rabins PV, Morrison A, Lyketsos C, Samus QM. Unmet needs of community-residing persons with dementia and their informal caregivers: findings from the

maximizing independence at home study. J Am Geriatr Soc. 2013;61:2087–95.

32. Johnston D, Samus QM, Morrison A, JLeoutsakos JS, Hicks K, Handel S, Rye R, Robbins B, Rabins PV, Lyketsos CG, Black BS. Identification of community-residing individuals with dementia and their unmet needs for care. Int J Geriatr Psychiatry. 2011;26:292–8.

33. Samus QM, Johnston D, Black BS, Hess E, Lyman C, Vavilikolanu A, Pollutra J, Leoutsakos KM, LGitlin LN, PRabins PV, Lyketsos CG. A multidimensional home-based care coordination intervention for elders with memory disorders: the maximizing independence at home (MIND) pilot randomized trial. Am J Geriatr Psychiatr. 2014;22:398–414.

34. Tanner JA, Black BS, Johnston D, Hess E, Leoutsakos JM, Gitlin LN, Rabins PV, Lyketsos CG, Samus QM. A randomized controlled trial of a community-based dementia care coordination intervention: effects of mind at home on caregiver outcomes. Am J Geriatr Psychiatr. 2015;23:391–402.

35. Boltz M, Capezuti E, Bowar-Ferres S, et al. Changes in the geriatric care environment associated with NICHE (nurses improving Care for Health System Elders). Geriatr Nurs. 2008;29:176–85.

36. Leff B, Burton L, Mader SL, et al. Hospital at home: feasibility and outcomes of a program to provide hospital-level care at home for acutely ill older patients. Ann Intern Med. 2005;143:798–808.

37. Branowicki PM, Vessey JA, Graham DA, McCabe MA, Clapp AL, Blaine K, O'Neill MR, Gouthro JA, Snydeman CK, Kline NE, Chiang VW, Cannon C, Berry JG. Meta-analysis of clinical trials that evaluate the effectiveness of hospital-initiated post discharge interventions on hospital readmission. J Healthc Qual. 2017;39(6):354–66. https://doi.org/10.1097/JHQ.0000000000000057.

38. Fox MT, Sidani S, Persaud M, Tregunno D, Maimets I, Brooks D, O'Brien K. Acute care for elders components of acute geriatric unit care: systematic descriptive review. J Am Geriatr Soc. 2013;61:939–46.

39. Ronneikko JK, Makela M, Jamsen EA, Huntala H, Finne-Soveri H, Noro A, Valvanne JN. Predictors for unplanned hospitalization of new homecare clients. J Am Ger Soc. 2017;65:407–14.

40. Dean KB, Hatfield LA, Jena AB, Cristman D, Flair M, Kator K, Nudd G, Grabowski DC. Preliminary data on a care

coordination program for home care recipients. J Am Geriatr Soc. 2016;64:1900–3.

41. www.nursinghomequalitycampaign.org. Accessed 17 Nov 2017.
42. Rosland AM, Nelson K, Sun H, Dolan ED, Maynard C, Bryson C, Stark R, Shear JM, Kerr E, Fihn SD, Schectman G. The patient-centered medical home in the Veterans Health Administration. Am J Manag Care. 2013;19(7):e263–72.
43. Moore AB, Krupp JE, Dufour AB, et al. Improving transitions to postacute care for elderly patients using a novel video–conferencing program: ECHO–care transitions. Am J Med. 2017;130:1199–204.
44. Rand Corporation. The evolving role of emergency departments in the United States, 2013. https://www.rand.org/content/dam/rand/pubs/research_reports/RR200/RR280/RAND_RR280.pdf. Accessed 17 Nov 2017.
45. Stevens M, Hastings SN, Markland A, Hwang U, Hung W, Vandenberg A, Bryan W, Cross D, Powers JS, McGwin G, Fattouh N, Ho W, Clevenger C, Vaughan C. Enhancing quality of provider practices for older adults in the emergency department (EQUiPPED). J Am Geriatr Soc. 2017;65(7):1609–14. https://doi.org/10.1111/jgs.14890.
46. Camden Coalition. http://healthcarehotspotting.com/wp/intro-duction/. Accessed 17 Nov 2017.
47. Sinhal SL. Living longer living well. Report to Ministry of Health and Long Term Care. 2012. http://www.health.gov.on.ca/en/common/ministry/publications/reports/seniors_strategy/. Accessed 17 Nov 2017.
48. Sinhal SL. (unpublished data) from Insights gained from the development of a community paramedicine program in Canada. Abstract presented at the 21st World Congress of Geriatrics and Gerontology, 2017. p. 49. https://academic.oup.com/DocumentLibrary/GERONI/01_GERONI_igx004.pdf. Accessed 17 Nov 2017.

Chapter 6
Educating New Healthcare Providers for the Twenty-First Century

Abstract Healthcare providers are members of the larger society and will be profoundly affected by the value-based transformation of health care. The healthcare workforce of the twenty-first century must be capable of managing increasingly complex patient populations utilizing new care models. It must foster the skills to work collaboratively in inter-professional teams supplied with technological and system supports. Healthcare providers must also be able to work collaboratively with patients in a shared effort to promote better health.

The Landscape

Value-based transformation in health care will refocus the training of healthcare providers. In addition to medical knowledge, clinicians of the future need to be fluent in the new language and concepts of value-based healthcare delivery. Efficient administration and medical care with markets rewarding quality and better patient outcomes will replace volume-based services. Transparent value-based insurance design incentivizes patient choices for higher quality treating clinicians and hospitals, and imposes increased personal health responsibility for cost of care and adoption of healthier lifestyles and adherence to effective treatments. Administrative tools and information technology that reduce

© Springer International Publishing AG, part of
Springer Nature 2018
J. S. Powers, *Value Driven Healthcare and Geriatric Medicine*,
https://doi.org/10.1007/978-3-319-77057-4_6

costs and ensure healthy competition will be important components of the healthcare landscape. Healthcare markets will drive outcome-based practice. Health plans will demand demonstration of clinical effectiveness while monitoring provider efficiency and outcome-based performance targets. There will be consequences to patients and providers for overspending [1, 2].

New healthcare professionals will need to contribute to the aims of value-based health care: better alignment of healthcare cost inflation with overall economic growth while ensuring access to appropriate evidence-based services for all. Clinician participation is critical as payment and delivery systems are transformed to consistently produce better care coordination and better outcomes at lower costs. The healthcare environment will foster more accountability and demonstrated effectiveness for care and services in terms of outcomes and safety. It will also involve more patient engagement, shared decision-making, and transparency in public reporting of quality and cost of care.

Educational Strategy

Healthcare practitioners of the twenty-first century must deliver care that is patient centered, of high quality, and effective [3]. They must be educated regarding new healthcare models, and value-based healthcare principles [4]. We must modernize healthcare delivery skills as well as train the workforce for the twenty-first-century healthcare in biomedical science [5, 6].

The healthcare workforce of the twenty-first century must be adept at managing increasingly complex patient populations, particularly as patients live longer and the burden of chronic disease continues to increase. We must align healthcare training to meet the nation's changing health needs and provide opportunities to foster the skills to work collaboratively in interdisciplinary team equipped with technological advances [6].

We needed an educational strategy fostering inter-professional teamwork. Team-based care is the future of health care and requires leadership and a highly functioning team of physicians, nurses, pharmacists, and specialists who understand the new healthcare system and its journey from volume to value, and appreciate the cultural heavy lifting that is going to be needed. The role of the physician will be to coach and support the work of each healthcare professional to function at the top of their scope of practice. The effective interdisciplinary team of the future will be highly interactive and focused on coordination of care, quality, and patient-centered care. Inter-professional education needs to be introduced in both undergraduate and graduate medical education in order to effect this cultural change.

Healthcare providers and healthcare organizations need to have competencies which equip them to survive and excel in a new transformational healthcare environment. They need information and training in governance, culture, leadership, policy development, and provider accountability. They must also be adept at including patients in decision-making processes that are aligned with value-based objectives. They need the ability to access longitudinal patient resources and evidence-based mechanisms for management of financial performance risk, and they need to establish provider networks and mechanisms to distribute shared savings payments. They will need the capacity to assess and implement products and platforms processing healthcare data. They will need timely access to reliable, key, actionable data for longitudinal patient management as well as analytics to evaluate interventions. They will need the ability to assess patient needs for chronic disease management and to navigate the health system to target strategies with specific resources using validated, risk-impact assessment tools (Table 6.1) [7].

Healthcare providers will also need longitudinal and interactive team care experiences with well-defined team member roles and responsibilities to foster continuity of care, access to well-targeted community-based social services, and reliable straightforward sharing of data across sites of care. They will

TABLE 6.1 Healthcare organizational competencies	• Governance and culture
	• Financial readiness
	• Health information technology
	• Patient risk assessment
	• Care coordination

TABLE 6.2 ACGME Core Competencies	• Patient care
	• Medical knowledge
	• Practice-based learning and improvement
	• Systems-based practice
	• Professionalism
	• Interpersonal skills and communication

need impact measurements on quality improvement programs and ability to make adjustments to processes of care. Healthcare providers of the future will need the capacity to help achieve individual patient's goals as expressed in their values, preferences, needs, and resultant care plans. Patients need to be heard, understood, and involved in their care.

Many medical trainees are obtaining additional business degrees or informatics skills to complement their medical training. They are aware that leadership positions of the future will need new skills to guide value-based transformation. The strength of physician leadership in health care is related to their clinical experience. It is that clinical focus which makes healthcare systems relevant to patient care. The High Value Healthcare Campaign of the American College of Physicians applies to trainees as well as practicing physicians, instilling value-based principles as basic clinical precepts early in their careers [8]. These new educational strategies complement and enhance the traditional six Accreditation Council for Graduate Medical Education (ACGME) Core Competencies [9] (Table 6.2).

Healthcare changes in progress will determine the job descriptions of geriatricians. Geriatric principles are likely to define mainstream healthcare practices as the care of older adults permeates the healthcare system and accounts for a disproportionate share of the costs [10]. A survey performed during the 2016 annual meeting of the DW Reynolds Educational Foundation included 115 geriatric educators and identified five future roles/job titles of geriatricians with implications for training beyond the skills required to care for older adults and their families (Table 6.3). Educators must be prepared to eliminate outdated expectations, incorporate critical elements and job skills associated with technology such as virtual visits, use big data analytics and prognostic tools, exhibit leadership skills and roles, work within and lead inter-professional teams, and be expert consultants and educators [11].

Collaborative practice models are being studied and promoted at the National Center for Inter-professional Practice and Education at the University of Minnesota. This public-private partnership provides leadership, evidence, and resources on inter-professional education and collaborative practice as a way to enhance the experience of health care, improving population health, and reducing overall cost of care to transform healthcare delivery [12] (Table 6.4).

A value-based care refocusing of ACGME Core Competencies (Table 6.2) tailored to primary care and inter-

TABLE 6.3 Geriatrician job roles

Complexivist—apply the latest best practices to inform care of medically complex patients

Consultant—support primary and specialist geriatric care utilizing new models of care

Health system leader and innovator—leading inter-professional teams, hospitals, and systems caring for geriatric populations

Functional preventionist—using data and prognostics to create preventive care models and monitor performance

Educator—designing geriatric medical education curricula applicable to all healthcare providers

TABLE 6.4 Goals of the National Center for Inter-professional Practice and Education

1. Care is patient centered, of high quality, and effective

2. Inter-professional teamwork

3. Coordination of care

4. Experiences in undergraduate and graduate medical
   education

professional team practice models could enhance the competencies in the following unique ways:

Patient care—experience in providing a team model of continuity of care, counseling, and preventive services for patients and families. Advocacy for models of care that are effective, and targeting of patients for appropriate interventions.

Medical knowledge—focusing on evidence-based primary care, prevention, screening, health promotion, chronic disease management, and health outcomes. Knowledge of prognosis, costs, and benefits of procedures.

Practice-based learning and improvement—participation in practice-based chronic disease management, setting and achieving quality care indicators, analyzing performance data.

Systems-based practice—supporting patients and families through transitions from hospital and nursing home back to home, facilitating home health care and other community-based services, development of medical neighborhoods with specialty physicians supporting chronic disease. Management models—participation in accountable care organizations, physician input to health systems performance.

Professionalism—developing collaborative models of care with other healthcare professionals particularly nurse practitioners and physician assistants, learning new physician management and consultative and collaborative roles and relationships to support delivery models with other healthcare professionals, focused on improved health outcomes.

Interpersonal skills and communication—developing team-based care models will take effort to overcome established physician incentives and practice styles influenced by fee-for-service models.

Establishing billing provider roles for advanced-practice nurses and physician assistants at teaching hospitals will also be challenging. Protocols to treat the majority of illnesses will need to be adapted and periodically updated [13]. There will be initial salary costs, care manager positions, and non-billable team meeting time that will need to be covered. Space for care managers, team meetings, and conferences will need to be accommodated. New practice roles for physicians as collaborators and advisors will need to be promoted with medical students and residents exposed early in their training, as future leaders of inter-professional teams, to promote productivity and satisfaction of all healthcare professionals in an autonomy-supportive fashion [14, 15]. Team-based care providers will also be expected to be knowledgeable about referral to community resources and how to support caregivers, and their training will need to prepare them for these roles.

Overuse is a major problem affecting the US healthcare system. An estimated one-third of care delivered in the United States is considered wasteful by the National Academy of Medicine. Even if overuse does not result in direct patient harm, evaluating the case for low-value care can still be instructive and offers opportunities to improve healthcare delivery in the future, as low-value care ultimately reduces availability of resources for other patients. As evidence increases about the harms from healthcare overuse, physicians have a professional obligation to reduce these events in both an individual patient level and across healthcare systems.

Overuse that results in clinical harm is a problem that should not be ignored by the safety community. Framing overuse through the lens of patient safety highlights it as an issue that affects the most important clinical outcomes for patients and clinicians. A patient safety infrastructure provides a mechanism for bringing overuse to attention and reducing its most harmful examples. Despite attention to overuse there are challenges to addressing overuse have been developed and validated [16].

References

1. Lewin JC, Atkins GL, McNeely L. The elusive past to healthcare sustainability. JAMA. 2013;310:1669–70.
2. Kocher R, Emanuel EJ, DeParle NM. The affordable care act and the future of clinical medicine: the opportunities and challenges. Annals Int Med. 2010;153:536–9.
3. Institute of medicine. Best care at lower cost: the path to continuously learning healthcare in America. Washington, DC: National academies press; 2012.
4. Rowe JW, Fulmer T, Fried L. Preparing for better health and health care for an aging population. JAMA. 2016;316:1643–4. https://doi.org/10.1001/jama.2016.12335.
5. Kruse J. Fragmentation in US medical education, research, and practice: the need for system wide defragmentation. Fam Med. 2013;45:54–7.
6. Lipstein SH, Kellermann AL, Berkowitz B, et al. Workforce for 21st-century health and health care: a vital direction for health and health care. Washington, DC: National Academy of Medicine; 2016.
7. McClellan MB, Leavitt MO. Competencies and tools to shift payments from volume to value. JAMA. 2016;316:1655–6.
8. American College of Physicians. Medical knowledge self-assessment program, 17. Philadelphia: American College of Physicians; 2015.
9. https://www.acgme.org/Portals/0/PDFs/ACGMEMilestones-CCC-AssesmentWebinar.pdf. Accessed 17 Nov 2017.
10. Tinetti M. Mainstream or extinction: can defining who we are save geriatrics? J Am Geriatr Soc. 2016;64:1400–4.
11. Simpson D, Leipzig RM, Sauvigne K, DW Reynolds Geriatrics Education Collaborative. The 2025 Big "G" geriatrician: defining job roles to guide fellowship training. J Am Geriatr Soc. 2017;65(10):2308–12. E pub ahead of print. https://doi.org/10.1111/jgs.14995.
12. The National Center for Interprofessional Practice and Education https://nexusipe.org/. Accessed 17 Nov 2017.

13. Paul S. Developing practice protocols for advanced practice nursing. AACN Clin Issues. 1999;10:343–55.
14. Deci EL, Eghvari H, Patrick BC, et al. Facilitating internalization: the self-determination. Perspective J Pers. 1994;62:119–42.
15. Powers JS, White S, Varnell L, et al. An autonomy supportive model of geriatric team function. Tennessee Medicine. 2000;93(8):295–7.
16. Lipitz-Snyderman A, Korenstein D. Reducing overuse–is patient safety the answer? JAMA. 2017;317(8):810–1.

Chapter 7
The Primary Care Dilemma

Abstract There is a great demand for primary care and outpatient services but a declining number of US medical trainees enter primary care each year. There is a mismatch between the need for care and service availability and society has hitherto exhibited a lackluster investment in the primary care infrastructure. Revitalizing primary care is crucial to value-based healthcare transformation.

Why Do We Have a Primary Care Problem?

The scope of primary care and its reach is huge. Geriatrics is in many respects a primary care specialty. With general medicine, family practice, and pediatrics, it shares the family-centered approach to the care of vulnerable populations, and accessing community resources to support caregivers. Geriatrics focuses on health promotion, prevention, and healthy aging, in addition to frailty, hospitalized elderly, managing advanced disease processes, rehabilitation, and long-term care. Geriatrics shares additional similarities with other primary care fields in that the demand exceeds the supply of physician providers, the comparatively low reimbursement under many health plans, and its historic lack of ability to attract trainees.

In the United States there is a great demand for primary care and outpatient services, but a declining number of

© Springer International Publishing AG, part of   97
Springer Nature 2018
J. S. Powers, *Value Driven Healthcare and Geriatric Medicine*,
https://doi.org/10.1007/978-3-319-77057-4_7

medical trainees enter primary care each year. There are many reasons for this mismatch between the need for care and service availability. This includes the high cost of medical education and large debts incurred by physicians in training, generally poor reimbursement for primary care and its long hours, excessive administrative tasks, and low prestige given to primary care by hospitals, health systems, and specialty colleagues. There has been a widening income gap between generalist and specialists, with many specialists earning two or more times that of primary care colleagues [1]. Consequently, there is a long waiting list for primary care services. This demand has helped stimulate the growth of advanced practice nurses (APNs) and physician assistants (PAs) who can care for an estimated 80% of primary care conditions and function well in a team-based care model. In a value-based healthcare environment a team-based primary care model can provide a patient-centered medical home for primary care as well as geriatrics. This is a major opportunity for collaborative physician leadership roles for the healthcare team. This value-based model can be further augmented by the use of new technology to facilitate and enhance interactions with patients, family caregivers, and participating team members who need not all be physically present at the same location in order to effectively function as a team.

Predicting the Extent of Need for Primary Care

The aging of the population requires an increased amount of primary care and physician workforce generally. There has been an increase in the number of primary care shortage areas defined as a population-to-physician ratio greater than 3000–1. Many primary care physicians are nearing retirement age, and 25% greater than the age of 60. The American Association of Medical Colleges (AAMC) predicts that by 2025, demand for physicians will exceed supply by a range of 46,100–90,400. The lower range estimate represents more aggressive delivery changes secondary to the rapid growth in non-physician clinicians and widespread adoption of new payment and delivery models such as Patient-Centered Medical Homes (PCMHs) and Accountable Care Organizations (ACOs). Total shortages in 2025 vary by specialty grouping as well as geographic location and include a shortfall of between 12,500 and 31,100 primary care physicians, and a shortfall of between 28,200 and 63,700 non-primary care physicians, including 5100–12,300 medical specialists, 23,100–31,600 surgical specialists, and 2400–20,200 other specialty physicians [2].

The physician shortage is particularly severe in rural areas and will persist under every likely scenario, including increased use of APNs and PAs, greater use of alternate settings such as retail clinics, delayed physician retirement, rapid changes in payment and delivery fueled by value-based purchasing, and other modeled scenarios. Addressing the shortage will require a multipronged approach, including innovation in care delivery; greater use of technology; improved, efficient use of all health professionals on the care team; and an increase in federal support for primary care training. No single solution will be sufficient on its own to resolve these predicted physician shortages. Because physician training can take up to a decade, a physician shortage in 2025 is a problem that needs to be urgently addressed now [2]. The shortage of primary care physicians is particularly concerning (Table 7.1) [3].

A primary care outpatient geriatrics practice is difficult to sustain in isolation. Many physicians see geriatric patients included in their mix of younger patients as part of a general medicine or family practice setting. An exclusively geriatric practice presents many challenges to the physician including the level of complexity and the need for ancillary support from social work, nursing, and pharmacy. Large healthcare systems have employed geriatricians to focus on the management of complex older adults, and may have disease management programs targeted for certain conditions such as hypertension, diabetes, and congestive heart failure which provide care management for selected patient populations. Alternative payment models (APMs) must include these

TABLE 7.1 Projected demand for primary care physicians—from Health Resources Service Administration (HRSA) [3]

Physician category	2010	2020
Total primary care physician demand (FTE)	212,500[a]	241,200
General[b]	164,400	187,300
Pediatrics	44,800	49,600
Geriatrics	3300	4300
Primary care physician supply	205,000	220,800
Supply and demand	(7500)	(20,400)

[a]National demand projections presented in this report assume that in 2010 the national supply of primary care physicians was adequate except for the approximately 7500 FTEs needed to de-designate the primary care health physician shortage areas
[b]This category includes general and family practice, and general internal medicine

value-added additional supports for programs targeting high-risk patients including older adults, patients with multi-morbidity, and those with advanced disease processes. The delivery of comprehensive primary care requires population-based payments aligned across payers to ensure adequate support for care delivery for all the patients in the practice.

Government and Organized Medicine Physician Responses

Society has undervalued primary care as reflected by a lack-luster investment in primary care infrastructure. Traditional fee-for-service (FFS) did not reimburse for non-face-to-face foundational service components of primary practice such as care coordination, transitions of care, and chronic care management. CMS has only recently recognized Evaluation and Management (E&M) codes for these conditions and for advance care planning, but the complexity of documentation and billing for the services has produced low uptake in billing practices.

The Council on Graduate Medical Education (COGME) has recommended that at least 40% of the physician workforce should practice primary care and that their salary should average no less than 70% of specialists' salaries [4]. In order to improve primary care access, safety net programs such as Community Health Centers (CHC) and Federally Qualified Health Centers (FQHC) were promoted as private nonprofit organizations providing primary health care in defined medically underserved areas. The centers receive federal grants from the Public Health Service Act to improve access for low-income, underserved, and vulnerable populations. In 2015 there were more than 9700 CHC sites serving 24 million patients [5]. Yet medical school graduates are shunning primary care in favor of more lucrative specialty careers as evidenced by direct correlation between mean overall specialty salary and US graduates' residency fill rates [6]. Congress has attempted a number of other inducements to attract patients into primary care offices and to promote primary care chronicled in Table 7.2 [7].

In 2006, in response to concerns of a future physician shortage, the Association of American Medical Colleges (AAMC) recommended a 30% increase in US medical school enrollment by 2015. Using the first-year enrollment of 16,488 students in 2002 as a baseline, a 30% increase would produce 21,434 first-year medical students enrolling by 2015, an increase of 4946 students. The percent of medical schools that were planning at least one initiative to increase student interest in primary care specialties rose from 49% in 2009 to 75% in 2010, and has remained above 70% in subsequent surveys. The survey results suggest that first-year medical school enrollment in 2019–2020 will reach 21,304 — a 29.2% increase over the 2002–2003 level and only 130 positions shy of the 30% target [8]. However, predictions based on specialty training data trends and 2017 postgraduate match results suggest that only 23% of physicians beginning residency will become generalists and 77% will specialize, with

TABLE 7.2 Federal efforts to promote primary care

• Low-interest loan programs for medical students pursuing primary care

• National Health Service Corps (NHSC) scholarship/loan payback program to recruit primary care clinicians to underserved areas

• Investments in Teaching Health Center Graduate Medical Education (GME) program (THCGME)—targeting primary care residency program expansion and increasing the number of primary care residency physicians and community-based training programs

• Enhancement to Title VII programs through the US Public Health Service Act to provide grants to fund training programs for primary care students, residents, faculty, and academic units

• Technical changes to the Medicare GME support program to permit increased funding to community-based primary care residency programs through an allocation of unfilled residency physicians redistributed to primary care

• Comprehensive Primary Care Plus (CPC+), a national advanced primary care medical home model to strengthen primary care through regionally based multi-payer payment reform and care delivery transformation

no progress toward the COGME goal of a workforce of 40% generalists [9].

CPC+ is an advanced APM that includes two primary care practice tracks with incrementally advanced care delivery requirements and payment options to meet the diverse needs of primary care practices. This 5-year program began Round 1 in 2017 and includes 2850 primary care practices. Round 2 began in 2018 in selected states. CPC+ is designed to strengthen primary care through a multi-payer model to ensure that the practices have approximately 50% or more of their current revenue generated by Medicare and other payers in the model. As a public–private partnership, all partners agree to support participating practices to make substantial changes in care delivery including patient access and continuity; care management for high-risk, high-need patients; engaging patients and caregivers; focusing on preventive care and population health; and increased comprehensive management and coordination of care [10, 11]. CPC+ payment for Medicare includes (1) two options for a non-visit-based, risk-adjusted, care management fee for attributed Medicare FFS beneficiaries paid quarterly in advance; (2) FFS reimbursement; and (3) a performance-based incentive payment. Early data suggests that many practices have achieved improvements in the delivery of primary care, with an alignment in delivery of care with these supportive learning and payment strategies.

Non-physician Approaches

As of 2017, 22 states, the District of Columbia, and the Veterans Administration allow full practice authority to APNs (no physician supervision required) [12] and PA's desire to achieve that same autonomy, with full practice authority currently granted in Michigan. There are approximately 106,000 APNs, of which 56,000 (52%) practice in primary care fields, and 70,000 PAs, of which 30,000 (43%) are in primary care fields [13]. The combined number of primary care APNs and PAs approximates 42% of the size of the current primary care physician workforce. Approximately 15,000 APNs [14] and 6776 PAs [15] are trained yearly in the United States. The growth of these primary care providers could help offset the need for primary care services traditionally filled by physicians.

A FFS payment system conflicts with collaborative care models. It inhibits team-based care and puts other providers, including APNs and PAs in competition with physicians. Some state medical societies continue to argue over the degree of supervision required and the authority to regulate the scope of practice of nonphysician providers.

The non-face-to-face coordination of care requirements and administrative time burden imposed on primary care providers amounts to 1–2 h for each hour of direct patient care, and is unsustainable [16]. The current burden of documentation related to the clinical encounter is imposed by billing requirements, quality reporting metrics, and justification for test ordering and services. Required documentation needs to be reduced and streamlined. Requirements to ensure that physicians perform and document unnecessary elements of care to justify billing codes but which do not contribute to good medical care should be eliminated. Payers must also develop a more efficient pre-approval process for tests, medications, services, and procedures.

Health promotion is a vital new direction for health care. This broad area includes partnerships with patients to promote responsibility for better health and well-being. System strategies for better health need to continue throughout the life course, addressing social determinants of health and health disparities, and prepare for better health and health care for an aging population. Chronic disease prevention and modification begin with tobacco use cessation, physical activity, good nutrition, and improving access to effective care for people who have mental health and substance-use disorders, thus advancing the health of communities and populations [17].

An Integrated Approach

Consider team-based health care as a primary care track solution—a blueprint for primary care transformation. New roles for physicians are the future in advanced APMs. Population-focused health care could advance the primary care situation. If the inclusion of the primary care healthcare professional provides value-added content to the quality and cost savings of the healthcare organization, primary care will be valued among the services for which the plan is accountable.

Physician team leaders must keep informed and solicit ideas and suggestions on how to improve the work unit, facilitate professional development of other team members, and acknowledge the individual contributions and achievements of each healthcare professional. To effectively facilitate professional development, the physician leader must recognize the aspect of work most professionally rewarding for each of the team members and provide coaching, mentorship, and opportunities for individuals to gain experience and successfully engage in these activities.

It is increasingly common for healthcare teams to be non-hierarchical. Healthcare team members assume leadership roles in different aspects of healthcare encounters. Consider these models for reenergizing primary care (Table 7.3).

Proven approaches to process implementation must be employed to improve workflow. Primary care-coordinated care must meet patient expectations and needs (Table 7.4). For some primary care services it may be possible to substitute phone, e-mail, and telehealth for live visits.

In a new primary care world, we must identify barriers to care and create plans to address these barriers. Easier access improves compliance. More frequent proactive contact with high-risk patients is an important care management technique. Patient-centered team members can share team report

TABLE 7.3 New models of primary care delivery [18]

- Team-based care with members functioning at the top of their scope (role)

- Reduce appointment backlog, carve out slots for urgent visits, reduce no-shows, and utilize phone visits when exam is unneeded

- Increased use of non-appointment care using protocols to develop and delegate tasks

- Offer same-day appointments including nursing visits, expanded team visits, and urgent visits

- Shared medical appointments for interdisciplinary evaluations, disease-specific group visits, and collaborative consultations with other colleagues

TABLE 7.4 Attributes of the patient-centered medical home

Access—Same-day appointments, shared medical appointments, non-appointment care

Care management and coordination—focus on high-risk patients, improved care for prevention and for chronic disease, improved transitions between the patient-centered medical home, inpatient, specialty care, and post-acute care

Practice redesign—redesign team member roles and tasks, enhance communication and teamwork, improve the processes of work during the visit as well as non-visit work

metrics which influence Physician Compare and use a dashboard as a care coordination tool. Dashboards and protocols are innovative ways to improve outcomes as well as provide real-time information that matters to the patient as well as the healthcare team. Improved electronic health record (EHR) user interfaces could deliver data that actually helps providers deliver better care with less effort and frustration. Interoperability between EHRs, such as utilizing the Fast Healthcare Inter-operability Resources (FHIR) framework and associated apps, would also facilitate transfer of care between institutions and providers.

It is unrealistic to think that every primary care team can have all support services available for every patient at all times. Efficiency requires consolidation of resources and a decreased number of steps to task completion, but conversely requires increased knowledge and capabilities of each team member. High-risk, high-need patients can be better managed utilizing expanded team members including social workers, pharmacists, and dietitians, on a "just-in-time" basis, perhaps even virtually. Artificial intelligence (AI) applied to EHR extraction and identification of at-risk patients can be value added, helping to guide team members to focus on appropriate patients.

In the patient-centered medical home, the roles of healthcare professionals are critical (Table 7.5).

Plan, Do, Study, Act (PDSA) cycles, originally described by Deming of Bell Laboratories (Table 7.6), are a good way to

TABLE 7.5 Roles of the primary care team members

RN—main point of contact, population management, utilizing data resources, coordinating care especially during high-risk transitions, functions as the care manager

LPN—supervision and delegation by the RN or PCP including focused assessments, health screenings, preventive procedures, health coaching, rooms the patient and assists the provider

Clerical associate—initial point of contact and patient advocate, customer service professional, handoff for communications, coordinates information, manages scheduling and recall

Provider—physician, nurse practitioner, physician's assistant-scheduled clinic visits, walk-in urgent visits, group visits, CBT visits, e-mail, team leadership in consultation, midlevel collaboration

TABLE 7.6 PDSA cycles

Plan—plan the test for observation, including a plan for collecting data, state the objective of the test

Do—try out the test on a small scale, document problems and observations

Study—check—analyze the data, compare the data to previous experience, and reflect on what was learned

Act—refine the change based on what was learned from the test, determining what modification should be made, and develop a plan for the next test

introduce quality improvement into primary care. Deciding on a topic important to the practice and implementing any change can help the team work collectively to achieve common goals.

Topics for PDSA cycles could include messaging/communications, analysis of effectiveness of care management, reducing appointments or waiting time, facilitation of workflow, medication reconciliation, or other topics of concern to the practice identified on review of operations data. A PDSA

TABLE 7.7 PDSA strategic work chart

Stage	Description	Steps
Plan	What is the goal?	What is the strategy?
	1.	1.
	2.	2.
	3.	3.
Do	Aim for small successes	Initiate (pilot), observe responses
	1.	1.
	2.	2.
	3.	3.
Study	Check outcomes	Reflect on lessons learned
	1.	1.
	2.	2.
	3.	3.
Act	Refine the goal	Modify the strategy, consider new resources
	1.	1.
	2.	2.
	3.	3.

work chart is one way to discuss quality improvement with staff and to operationalize the process (Table 7.7).

The concept of SMART Processes [19] is another strategy to engage staff collaboratively to enhance performance toward defined quality metrics (Table 7.8). Review of operations data can identify gaps in care. Performing a strategic review and planning for change, and selecting an intervention that is appropriate to the practice, are highly recommended exercises. Interventions should have a specific focus, have a measurable outcome, be practical and attainable, be relevant

TABLE 7.8 SMART processes

Specific
Measurable
Attainable
Relevant
Time bound

to the goals of the institution, and be time bound to the institution's quality improvement cycle. Analyzing the results and refining the change lead to another PDSA cycle.

Administrative tasks take time and focus away from other clinically important activities of physicians. A collaborative practice model can permit review and delegation of tasks to different team members appropriate to their skill level, freeing the clinician to focus on more clinically relevant duties [20].

New models for primary care have been demonstrated to increase patient access and create efficiencies for the physician. Examples include telehealth, group appointments, video telehealth virtual visits, and Internet weight loss programs [21–24]. In addition to efficiency, these collaborative models enhance access by keeping patients close to their home.

Regulatory Approach

Medicare Graduate Medical Education (GME) financing is the largest public investment in healthcare workforce development and with two-thirds of nearly $10 billion manual funding going to the 200 hospitals training the largest number of residents. Despite this massive funding level, the physician workforce continues to face critical shortages in specific specialties and locations, most of which are minimally served by the graduates of those 200 hospitals. As a result, Medicare GME-funded institutions face increased scrutiny and calls for greater accountability. A secondary analysis of the AMA Physician Master File indicates that only 25% of physicians in training between 2006 and 2008 were in primary care 5 years post-residency. The broad definition of primary care included pediatrics, general medicine, family practice, psychiatry, OB/GYN, and general surgery. As early as 1965 and as recently as 2011 advisory bodies have recommended that GME be more accountable to the public's needs. These institutions include the National Academy of Medicine, the ACGME, and the Josiah Macy Jr. Foundation [25]. The population demands more primary care and primary care is a major contributor to value-based healthcare. As medical education is publicly funded, it is highly probable that GME will be held accountable to society's needs.

Some have suggested dividing GME accountability into three specific domains: (1) guarantee individual trainee competence to meet the needs of individual patients and the public at large; (2) require training in diverse clinical settings to demonstrate safe high-quality, high-value patient-centered care; and (3) GME programs must produce a physician workforce of the appropriate size, specialty mix, and geographic distribution to meet the needs of the public [26]. The American College of Physicians agrees that the concept of a performance-based GME payment system is an idea that is worth exploring. Such a system should be thoughtfully developed and considered in a deliberate way to ensure that payment of Medicare GME funds to hospitals and training programs is tied to the nation's healthcare workforce needs. Payments should be used to meet policy goals to ensure an adequate supply, specialty mix, and site of training [27]. A competitive peer review process similar to the NIH grant process and lifting GME funding caps for needed primary care resident positions and training programs are possible strategies for change.

Additional strategies to enhance primary care could include an emphasis in developing primary care faculty, recruiting primary care-oriented students, and enhancing primary care curricula and training experiences to make longitudinal care of patients relevant and compelling as a profession. Primary care training for new providers must also include confidence building and leadership skills, cultivate independence, and demonstrate how to build collaborative team relationships. The development of a longitudinal mentoring relationship with a primary care physician can be critical for role modeling and to demonstrate a successful primary care career. Primary care must be presented as the complex and interesting specialty that it is [7]. Trainees need focused learning of outpatient primary care which is just as demanding and difficult as inpatient medicine. Primary care is associated with fewer adverse effects, medical errors, complications, excessive testing, more preventive care, and reduced disparities among populations—all of the things that are so important in value-based purchasing [28]. It is also imperative that we promote the value proposition of primary care as associated with more equitable distribution of health in the population, and improved health and quality of life for individuals and populations.

References

1. Bodenheimer T, Berenson RA, Rudolf P. The primary care–specialty income gap: Why it matters. Ann Intern Med. 2007;146:301–6.
2. AAMC Physician supply and demand through 2025: Key findings. https://www.aamc.org/download/426260/data/physiciansupplyanddemandthrough2025keyfindings.pdf. Accessed 17 Nov 2017.
3. HRSA Projecting the supply and demand for primary care practitioners through 2020. https://bhw.hrsa.gov/sites/default/files/bhw/nchwa/primarycarebrief.pdf. Accessed 17 Nov 2017.
4. Council on Graduate Medical Education Twentieth Report: Advancing primary care. December 2010. https://www.hrsa.gov/advisorycommittees/bhwadvisory/co%20gme/Reports/twentiethreport.pdf. Accessed 17 Nov 2017.
5. National Association of Community Health Centers (NACHC) United States Health Center fact sheet. http://www.nachc.org/wp-content/uploads/2017/03/US17.pdf#5. Accessed 17 Nov 2017.
6. Ebell MH. Future salary and US residency fill rate revisited. JAMA. 2008;300:1131–2.

7. Klink K. Incentives for physicians to pursue primary care in the ACA era. Am Med Assoc J Ethics. 2015;17:637–46.
8. AAMC Results of the 2014 medical school enrollment survey https://members.aamc.org/eweb/upload/Results%20of%20 the%202014%20Medical%20School%20Enrollment%20 Survey.pdf. Accessed 17 Nov 2017.
9. Dalen JE, Ryan KJ, Alpert JS. The 2017 match and the future US workforce. Am J Med. 2018;131:2–4.
10. Centers for Medicare and Medicaid Services. Comprehensive primary care plus https://innovation.cms.gov/initiatives/comprehensive-primary-care-plus. Accessed 3 Nov 2017.
11. Sessums LL, Conway PH. Saving primary care. JAMA Intern Med. 2017;117:1560–1.
12. Simmons School of Nursing Where Can Nurse Practitioners Work Without Physician Supervision? https://onlinenursing.simmons.edu/nursing-blog/nurse-practitioners-scope-of-practice-map/. Accessed 3 Nov 2017.
13. Agency for Healthcare Research and Quality The number of nurse practitioners and physician assistants practicing primary care in the United States. Primary care workforce facts and stats #2 https://www.ahrq.gov/research/findings/factsheets/primary/pcwork2/index.html. Accessed 3 Nov 2017.
14. American Association of Nurse Practitioners. https://www.aanp.org/press-room/press-releases/161-press-room/2014-press-releases/1675-2015-nurse-practitioner-ranks-surge-to-205-000-nearly-doubling-over-past-decade. Accessed 3 Nov 2017.
15. Hooker RS, Cawley JF, Everett CM. Predictive modeling the physician assistant supply: 2010–2025. Public Health Rep. 2011;126(5):708–16.
16. Sinsky C, Colligan L, Li L, Prgomet M, Reynolds S, Goeders L, Westbrook J, Tutty M, Blike G. Allocation of physician time in ambulatory practice: a time and motion study in 4 specialties. Ann Intern Med. 2016;165:753–60.
17. Taylor LA, Coyle CE, Ndumele C, et al. Leveraging the social determinants of health: what works? Boston, MA: Blue Cross Blue Shield of Massachusetts Foundation; 2015. http://bluecrossfoundation.org/sites/default/files/download/publication/Social_Equity_Report_Final.pdf. Accessed 17 Nov 2017.
18. Improving primary care. Strategies and tools for a better practice Bodenheimer, Thomas, Grumbach, Kevin (UCSF Primary Care). New York: McGraw-Hill; 2007. ISBN paperback 9780071447386.

19. Doran GT. There's a S.M.A.R.T. Way to write management's goals and objectives. Management review. AMA Forum. 1981;70(11):35–6.

20. Erikson SM, Rockwern B, Koltov M, McLean RM, for the medical practice in quality committee of the American College of physicians. Putting patients first by reducing administrative tasks and healthcare: A position paper of the American College of physicians. Ann Intern Med. 2017;166:659–61.

21. Berman M, Fenaughty A. Technology and managed care: patient benefits of telemedicine in a rural health care network. Health EconHealth Econ. 2005;14:559–73.

22. Hailey D, Roine R, Ohinmaa A. Systematic review of evidence for the benefits of telemedicine. J Telemed Telecare. 2002;8(suppl 1):1–30.

23. Lyles C. Seeing the effect of health care delivery innovation in the safety net. JAMA Intern Med. 2017;177:649–50.

24. Phelan S, Hagobian T, Brannen A, Hatley KE, Schaffner A, Munoz-Christian K, Tate DF. Effect of an Internet–based program on weight loss for low–income postpartum women. A randomized clinical trial. JAMA. 2017;317:2381–91.

25. Chen C, Petterson S, Phillips RL, Mullan F, Bazemore A, O'Donnell SD. Toward graduate medical education (GME) accountability: measuring the outcomes of GME institutions. Acad MedAcad Med. 2013;88:1267–80.

26. Baron RB. Can we achieve Public accountability for graduate medical education outcomes? Acad Med. 2013;88:1199–201.

27. American College of Physicians. Policy paper. 2011. Aligning GME policy with the Nation's health care workforce needs. Https://www.acponline.org/system/files/documents/advocacy/current_policy_papers/assets/gme_policy.pdf. Accessed 17 Nov 2017.

28. Starfield B, Shi L, Macinko J. Contribution of primary care to health systems and health. Milbank Q. 2005;83:457–502.

Chapter 8
Transitions of Care

Abstract Value-based purchasing requires healthcare systems to strategize by considering all elements of the continuum of care. Covered beneficiaries enrolled in the health system must be efficiently managed at each level of care and appropriate communication, acknowledgment, and respect for each component along the healthcare continuum are essential for optimum patient experience of care, quality performance, and value.

Scope of the Issue

Value-based purchasing requires healthcare systems to strategize to maximize efficiency and effectiveness by considering all elements of the continuum of care. Covered beneficiaries enrolled in healthcare systems must be efficiently managed at each level of care, and appropriate communication, acknowledgement, and respect for each component of the healthcare continuum are essential for optimum patient experience of care, outcome performance, and value [1–4]. Because the hospital is the major

© Springer International Publishing AG, part of
Springer Nature 2018
J. S. Powers, *Value Driven Healthcare and Geriatric Medicine*,
https://doi.org/10.1007/978-3-319-77057-4_8

component of a healthcare system and provides the most expensive services, it is natural to focus on acute care. However, neglecting other elements of care across about continuum puts performance objectives at risk, harms the patient experience of care, and increases cost. Value-based purchasing has forced administrators to consider cost avoidance as an important and critical part of the business plan. Cost avoidance is now a new cost center, essential to minimizing downside (loss) risk. This involves targeting appropriate sites of care for disease management programs, including post-acute care facilities and home and community-based services.

The US spends the most healthcare resources of any Organization for Economic Cooperation and Development (OECD) country, amounting to $9523 per capita (2014) [5]. For every dollar spent on health care, OECD countries spend two dollars on social services, compared to $0.50 for the United States [6], placing the United States far below many other countries in spending on home and community-based services (Fig. 8.1).

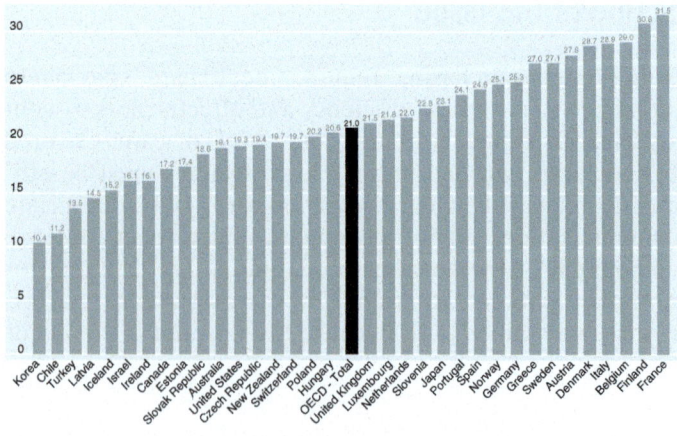

FIGURE 8.1 Social spending, public (OECD 2017) [7]

Models to Improve Transitions of Care

The cost of unplanned rehospitalizations to the Medicare program is estimated at over $12 billion yearly [8]. Beyond economic implications, suboptimal care transitions increase the risk of adverse events resulting from poor care coordination among providers and healthcare facilities. A work group convened by the Patient-Centered Outcomes Research Institute (PCORI) identified eight transitional care components and operational strategies to enhance transitional care, and analyzed how well the set aligned with real-world patient and caregiver experiences (Table 8.1).

For frail elderly patients, early readmission to hospital within 7 days of discharge to post-acute care facilities is associated with a shorter initial hospital length of stay. Admissions between 7 and 30 days are more common among patients with multiple comorbidities and exacerbations of advanced disease processes [10]. The National Transition of Care Coalition recommends shifting the discharge paradigm from *discharge from the hospital* to *transfer with continuous management*. Practice changes that could potentially impact readmission rates include hospitalist education regarding realistic post-acute care capabilities; emerging strategies to improve coordination, communication, and cooperation among healthcare professionals across healthcare settings; and maximizing stability of multiple comorbidities prior to discharge [11–14].

The Institute for Health Improvement (IHI) developed a National Healthcare Safety Network (NHSN) to help improve the coordination of care. In 2011 CMS launched the Community-based Care Transitions Program (CCTP). This program was designed to allow for testing of care models to improve transitions of Medicare beneficiaries from the inpatient hospital setting to other care settings, to improve the quality of care reducing readmissions for high-risk beneficiaries, and to document measurable savings to the Medicare program. Results from early implementation of the CCTP and intervention communities found that, compared with

TABLE 8.1 Transitions of care barriers identified by patients and families. *Modified from PECORI report* [9]

Category	Example	Strategy
Patient engagement	Lack of engagement	Comprehensive assessment
		Person-centered care
Caregiver engagement	Inadequate communication	Monitoring progress
		Provide caregiver resources
Complexity/ medication	Complex treatment regimens	Identify high-risk patients
Management	Reduce polypharmacy	
Patient education	Inadequate preparation	Address health literacy
Caregiver education	Gaps in services	Provide information
		Respect caregiver role
Patient and caregiver well-being	Multiple health/ social challenges	Recognize common concerns
		Provide caregiver resources
Care continuity	Poor continuity of care	Team communication
Accountability of clinician/team/ organization	Poor communication	Enhanced collaboration with referral sources

uninvolved communities, the all-cause 30-day rehospitalization and all-cause hospitalization rate declined [15]. Additionally, CMS has developed a national nursing home quality of care collaborative (NNHCC) with a focus on improving the quality of care and quality of life among nursing home residents by instilling quality and performance improvement practices and encouraging development of quality improvement projects in all long-term care facilities. CMS required the Quality Improvement Organizations (QIOs) to support the adoption of the Quality Assessment and Performance Improvement (QAPI) framework as part of the nursing home action plan. In 2014 the QIOs have expanded to regional quality improvement networks of contiguous states in order to share best practices in coordinate regional quality improvement efforts [16].

In a report of Medicaid accountable care organizations (ACO) models in Oregon and Colorado, standardized monthly expenditures for individual declined similarly in both states between 2010 and 2014, despite the adoption of very different models. Oregon's model was further associated with reductions of emergency department visits and preventable acute hospital admissions. The approach Oregon took developed coordinated care organizations that accepted full financial risk marked by global budgeting. Colorado on the other hand initiated Medicaid accountable care collaboratives which received fee-for-service payments with no downside financial risk [17].

The Eastern Virginia Care Transitions Partnership, a network of health systems with a total of 69 skilled nursing facilities, area agencies on aging, and physician group practices, achieved a 30-day hospital readmission rate reduction from 22 to 8% (2013–2015) utilizing a synergistic approach of targeting high-risk patients and utilizing care coaches (Coleman Transitions Program) [3] as part of a Medicare pilot demonstration (Kyle Allen, unpublished data).

Similarly in a VA transformational care demonstration project, a geriatric patient-centered medical home (Geri-PACT) [18] utilizing a nurse care manager for high-risk elderly patients with multiple comorbidities was able to reduce 30-day hospital readmissions from 20 to 6% (2011–2016). The Geri-PACT Team consists of the Geri-PACT provider geriatrician or geriatric nurse practitioner serving a population of approximately 800, a social worker, a clinical pharmacist, a licensed vocational nurse, and clerical staff, working as a coordinated unit delivering patient-centered assessments and managing medically complex and vulnerable elderly individuals. Patients and caregivers received frequent communications from the Geri-PACT Team including contact when hospitalized, and following discharge from hospital and post-acute care facilities (James Powers, unpublished data).

A novel videoconference program, Extension for Community Health Outcomes–Care Transitions (ECHO–CT), has recently been described, connecting an interdisciplinary hospital-based team with clinicians at skilled nursing facilities [19]. In this program a hospital-based team conferenced with clinicians at post-acute care facilities to discuss issues arising during transitions of care. Issues addressed include a summary of the hospital course, an update on the patient's current condition, a review of medications, and discussions related to treatment plans. Discussions of individual patients varied in duration from a few minutes up to 10 min depending on the medical complexity and post-discharge concerns that arose at the skilled nursing facility. The program has been found to reduce patient mortality, hospital readmission, skilled nursing facility length of stay, and 30-day healthcare costs. ECHO is based on the experience of disease-based specialty programs collaborating with community health providers [20], and has been duplicated at 94 academic and expert hubs in the United States and 16 other countries [21].

Older adults transferring from skilled nursing facilities (SNF) to home have significant risk for poor outcomes. The Connect–Home Transitional Care Program is a four-step transitional care process which includes procedures for staff in SNFs to interact on patient care teams to deliver transitional care. In step 1, staff, patients, and caregivers create a transition plan of care using a consistent template in the EMR by days 15–17 of the SNF stay. In step 2 staff convene a care plan meeting to set priorities, review plans, and educate patient and caregiver. In step 3, staff, patients, and caregivers implement the transition plan: medication reconciliation, final treatment plan orders, scheduled follow-up appointments, and fax medical records to community clinicians. In step 4, the SNF social worker telephones the patient and caregiver for follow-up on the care plan. This program appears to provide better preparedness for discharge and addresses more caregiver needs with fewer self-reported falls, emergency room visits, and hospitalizations [22].

Performance Objectives Drive Behavior

CMS is clear that performance objectives for health systems include adhering to quality reporting measures. This mandate constitutes a very important lever for behavioral change. It is unclear how healthcare systems will meet new inpatient and outpatient quality reporting metrics, but these regulations come with heavy financial penalties for noncompliance. Underperforming health systems also have a risk of loss of market share as competing institutions develop network affiliations with community referral resources to create ACOs. Healthcare systems are financially encouraged by CMS with higher reimbursement to participate in advanced alternative payment models (APMs) such as next-generation ACOs, Bundled Payment Care Initiatives (BCPIs), Comprehensive Primary Care Plus (CPC+), and Medicare Track 2 and 3 Shared Savings Programs (MSSPs). Outpatient APMs also include focused disease management programs, and physician payment models tied to quality targets. APMs all have different risk profiles and many require initial capital investment (Chap. 5).

The Veterans Health Administration (VA) is also transforming the culture of care in nursing homes, enhancing person-centered care, care transitions, and communication among care programs as part of its quality improvement program. The VA is responsible for managing nursing home patients at three levels of long-term care (LTC): Community Living Centers (CLC), State Veterans Homes (SVH), and contracted Community Nursing Homes (CNH). CLCs are facilities run and staffed by the VA, SVHs are constructed with joint VA-state support but are managed privately, and CNHs which are privately owned and operated provide care to veterans in the community. The VA surveys care to provide oversight and to optimize resident care in long-term care (LTC) facilities and spent $767 million in FY 2013 for contracted community nursing home care [23].

The benefits of the Acute Care for Elderly (ACE) Units include the reduction of iatrogenic complications and preservation of functional status [24]. Similarly, the Patient-Centered Medical Home (PCMH) model strives to manage patients across the continuum of care. These models can be projected to population needs with process standardization to reduce variation and to benefit healthcare systems. New tools to improve processes of care and to make care more age friendly include analyzing service components via focused patient-segmented matrices, creative use of technology to personalized care and create value (disruptive innovation), and interoperability of the electronic health record (EHR) with increased connectivity, both actual and virtual. The opportunity to extend the PCMH model to acute and long care may facilitate the process of care [25]. Fig. 8.2 demonstrates age-friendly principles and the PCMH applied to senior friendly hospitals.

When seniors are hospitalized they become vulnerable to unexpected challenges including hospital-acquired delirium and functional decline that complicate their ability to return

 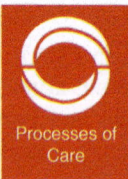  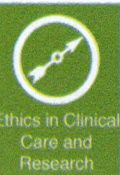 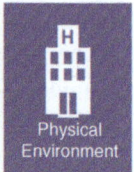

Figure 8.2 The senior-friendly hospital framework—geriatric principles applied to senior-friendly hospitals. Reproduced with permission from the Regional Geriatric Program of Toronto From http://seniorfriendlyhospitals.ca/about-sfh

to their place of residence. Organizations using the Senior Friendly Hospital Framework have found that careful attention to five healthcare organizational domains can improve outcomes over the continuum of care.

Organizational Support—In a senior-friendly hospital, leadership is committed to deliver an optimal experience for frail seniors as an organizational priority. This commitment empowers the development of human resources, policies and procedures, caregiving processes, and physical spaces that are sensitive to the needs of frail patients.

Demonstration of organizational support can include corporate and organizational commitment written into strategic plans or reported to hospital boards, formal quality improvement plans involving the advancement of senior-friendly hospital concepts, organizational support for inter-professional practice, and embedding senior-friendly principles in the planning and delivery of all clinical and nonclinical programs and services across the organization. The organization can also promote the development of clinical expertise and geriatrics by providing geriatric resources and champions for every patient care unit, training and mentorship to develop clinical skills and geriatrics, and senior sensitivity training for all clinical staff. The organization can also promote information and technology to support senior health care by analyzing aging-stratified patient experienced data to identify the unique needs of frail patients, and developing an integrated medical record and other processes to enhance interagency information sharing.

Processes of Care—In a senior-friendly hospital, care is designed from evidence and best practices that are mindful of physiology, pathology, and social science of aging and frailty. Care and service across the organization are delivered in a way that is integrated with the healthcare system and support transitions to the community.

Emotional and Behavioral Environment—In a senior-friendly hospital, care and service are provided in a way that is free of ageism and respects the needs of patients and their caregivers. This maximizes quality and satisfaction with the hospital experience.

Thoughtful attention is provided to the following elements consistent with the vulnerabilities of older adults and in a manner to create senior-friendly emotional and behavioral experience, including person-centered care, culture and diversity, safety, and prevention of elder abuse.

Ethics in Clinical Care and Research—In a senior-friendly hospital, care is provided in a way that protects the autonomy, choice, and diversity of the most vulnerable patients.

This includes meaningful consideration of the patient and family perspective regarding advance care planning and capacity and consent.

Physical Environment—In a senior-friendly hospital, the structures, spaces, equipment, and furnishings provide an environment that minimizes the vulnerabilities of frail patients, promoting safety, comfort, independence, and functional well-being.

The use of senior-friendly design resources in addition to accessibility and building code requirements supports cost-neutral implementation of physical design, purchasing, and maintenance activities for a physical environment that optimizes the safety and independence of frail populations.

The work ahead is clear. There remains a major effort to encourage health systems see the benefits of supporting care across the continuum, to share resources to enhance the individual care components and sites of care, to value each component contributing to outcomes of care, and to improve communication across the continuum. Development of patient-centered medical homes and disease management programs and creation of real partnerships with sharing of resources with other important contributors to the healthcare network are critical to supporting smooth transitions of care, minimizing cost, and maintaining patient outcome objectives for the healthcare systems (Table 8.2).

A meta-analysis of multicomponent quality improvement interventions to prevent hospital readmission suggests that interventions that engaged the general population and their caregivers may offer greater value to the health system [27].

TABLE 8.2 Transitions of care: models that work [26]

- Improve communication during transitions between providers, patients, and family caregivers

- Implement electronic health records that include standardized medication reconciliation elements

- Expand the role of pharmacists in transitions of care in respect to medication reconciliation

- Establish points of accountability for sending and receiving care, particularly for hospitalists, SNFists, primary care physicians, and specialists

- Increase the use of case management and professional care coordination

- Implement payment systems that align incentives

- Develop performance measures to encourage better transitions of care

Long-Term Care Insurance

The need for long-term care services at both institutional and community levels is growing exponentially. We need a comprehensive mechanism to pay for long-term care services, both skilled and unskilled, such as a voluntary, public, long-term care income option similar to social security. Few individuals are purchasing long-term care insurance on their own, and the cost is increasing. The American Association for Long Term Care Insurance estimates that only 8 million Americans have long-term care insurance, representing less than 20% of the over-65 population [28]. However, as the population ages, nearly all will need long-term care services, driving the demand for care in the community and home as well as institutional based care. The population of elderly over 65 is expected to comprise 77 million people by 2035. Estimates are that 6 out of 10 individuals will need long-term care sometime during their lifetime. Based on current estimates of the rate of long-term care this means that 17 million elderly Americans will be receiving long-term care in 2035. Some combination of public safety net programs, together with incentives for increased personal savings to purchase long-term care insurance, could provide viable policy solutions [29]. This would help broaden the risk pool with the goal of expanding insurance protection as well as secure the financing system for long-term care for the future [30].

References

1. Naylor MD, Brooten DA, Campbell RL, Maislin G, McCauley KM, Schwartz JS. Transitional care of older adults hospitalized with heart failure: a randomized, controlled trial. J Am Geriatr Soc. 2004;52:675–84.
2. Ouslander J, Lamb G, Tappan R, et al. Interventions to reduce hospitalizations from nursing homes: evaluation of the INTERACT II collaborative quality improvement project. J Am Geriatr Soc. 2011;59:745–53.
3. Coleman EA, Smith JD, Frank JC, Min S, Parry C, Kramer AM. Preparing patients and caregivers to participate in care delivered across settings: The care transitions intervention. J. Am Geriatr. Soc. 2004;42:1817–25.
4. Vasilevskis EE, Ouslander JG, Mixon AS, Bell SP, Jacobsen JM, Saraf AA, Markley D, Sponsler KC, Shutes J, Long EA, Kripalani S, Simmons SF, Schnelle JF. Potentially avoidable readmissions of patients discharged to post-acute care: perspectives of hospital in skilled nursing facility staff. J Am Ger Soc. 2017;65:269–76.
5. Centers for Disease Control, National Center for Health Statistics. Health, United States (2015) https://www.cdc.gov/nchs/fastats/health-expenditures.html. (overview- Tables 93-95) Accessed 17 Nov 2017
6. Bradley EH, Taylor LA. The American health care paradox: why spending more is getting us less. New York, NY: Public Affairs; 2013.
7. OCED (2017), Social spending (indicator). doi: https://doi.org/10.1787/7497563b-en Accessed 5 Oct 2017.
8. Medicare Payment Advisory Commission. A path to bundled payment around a rehospitalization. In: Report to the Congress: reforming the delivery system. Washington, DC; 2005. p. 83–103.

9. Patient Centered Outcomes Research Institute (PCORI) Transitional care workgroup meeting July 12, 2013 https://www.pcori.org/assets/2013/08/PCORI-Transitional-Care-Workgroup-April-2013-Meeting-Summary-071213.pdf. Accessed 25 Jan 2018.

10. Naylor MD, Shaid EC, Carpenter D, et al. Components of comprehensive and effective transitional care. J Am Geriatr Soc. 2017;65:1119–25.

11. Horney C, Capp R, Boxer R, Burke RE. Factors associated with early readmission among patients discharged to post-acute care facilities. J Am Geriatr Soc. 2017;65:1199–205.

12. Bradley EH, Curry L, Horwitz LI, et al. Contemporary evidence about hospital strategies for reducing 30-day readmissions: a national study. J Am Coll Cardiol. 2012;60:607–14.

13. Bradley EH, Curry L, Horwitz LI, et al. Hospital strategies associated with 30-day readmission rates for patients with heart failure. Circ Cardiovasc Qual Outcomes. 2013;6:444–50.

14. Figueroa JF, Joynt KE, Zhou X, Orav EJ, Jha AK. Safety-net hospitals face more barriers yet use fewer strategies to reduce readmissions. Med Care. 2017;55:229–35.

15. Brock J, Mitchell J, Irby K, et al. Association between quality improvement for care transitions in communities and rehospitalizations among Medicare beneficiaries. JAMA. 2013;309:381–91.

16. Mims AD, Pederson JC, Gold JA. Healthcare changes and the affordable care act: a physician call to action quality improvement organizations. In: Powers JS, editor. Healthcare changes and the affordable care act. Switzerland: Springer International Publishing; 2015. p. 13–31.

17. McConnell KJ, Renfro S, Chan BKS, et al. Early performance and Medicaid accountable care organizations. A comparison of Oregon and Colorado. JAMA Intern Med. 2017;177:538–45.

18. Department of Veterans Affairs, Veterans Health Administration. 2015. Patient aligned care team (Geri-PACT) handbook. Washington, DC. https://www.va.gov/vhapublications/ViewPublication.asp?pub_ID=3115. Accessed 17 Nov 2017.

19. Moore AB, Krupp JE, Dufour AB, et al. Improving transitions to postacute care for elderly patients using a novel video–conferencing program: ECHO–care transitions. Am J Med. 2017;130:1199–204.

20. Arora S, Thornton K, Jenkusky SM, Parish B, Scalentti JV, Project ECHO. Linking university specialist with rural and prison–based clinicians to improve care for people with chronic

hepatitis C in New Mexico. Public Health Rep. 2007;122(suppl 2):74–7.

21. Barash D. Tele–mentoring is creating global communities or practice in healthcare. Harv Bus Rev 2016. https://hbr.org/2016/11/tele-mentoring-is-creating-global-communities-of-practice-in-health-care. Accessed 20 Oct 2017.

22. Toles M, Colon-Emeric C, Naylor MD, Asafu-Adjei J, Hanson LC. Connect home: transitional care of skilled nursing facility patients and their caregivers. J Am Geriatr Soc. 2017;65:2322–8.

23. Veterans Health Administration, OIG, Office of Audits and Evaluations: Audit of the community nursing home program. March 29, 2013 No. 11-0031-160.

24. Fox MT, Sidani S, Persaud M, Tregunno D, Maimets I, Brooks D, O'Brien K. Acute care for elders components of acute geriatric unit care: systematic descriptive review. J Am Geriatr Soc. 2013;61:939–46.

25. Wong R. Geriatric program development in the future hospital. Abstract presented at the 21st World Congress of Geriatrics and Gerontology, 2017. p.78, Available at https://academic.oup.com/DocumentLibrary/GERONI/01_GERONI_igx004.pdf Senior Friendly Hospital toolkit at http://seniorfriendlyhospitals.ca/about-sfh. Accessed 17 Nov 2017.

26. National Transitions of Care Coalition, 2010. Improving transitions of care. http://www.ntocc.org/portals/0/pdf/resources/ntoccissuebriefs.pdf. Accessed 17 Nov 2017.

27. Nuckols TK, Keeler E, Mortobn S, et al. Economic evaluation of quality improvement interventions designed to prevent hospital readmission. A systematic review and meta-analysis. JAMA. 2017;177:975–85.

28. American Association for Long-term Care Insurance. Long-term care insurance fast facts. http://www.aaltci.org/long-term-care-insurance/learning-center/fast-facts.php. Accessed 17 Nov 2017.

29. Stevenson DG, Cohen MA, Tell EJ, Burwell B. The complementarity of public and private long–term care coverage. Health Aff (Millwood). 2010;29:96–101.

30. Cornell PY, Grabowski DC, Cohen M, Shi X, Stevenson DG. Medical underwriting in long-term care insurance: a conditions limited options for high risk consumers. Health Aff (Millwood). 2016;35:1494–503.

Chapter 9
Dual Eligibles: Challenges for Medicare and Medicaid Coordination

James S. Powers and Laura M. Keohane

Abstract The dual eligibles are low-income older adults and younger persons with significant disabilities who are enrolled in both the Medicare and Medicaid programs. This population depends heavily on the structure of healthcare financing, eligibility determination, and both federal and state funding. Changes in access and eligibility, and the disparity among states, could profoundly affect quality metrics and consequently the health of the dual-eligible population.

Scope of the Problem

The dual eligibles constitute the population of low-income older adults and younger persons with significant disabilities. All dual eligibles qualify for full Medicare benefits, but they differ in the amount of Medicaid benefits for which they are eligible. Approximately 88% are "full duals," who qualify for full benefits from both programs. The other 22% are "partial duals," who do not meet the eligibility requirements for full Medicaid benefits but qualify to have Medicaid pay some of the costs they incur under Medicare. Some 60% of dual eli-

© Springer International Publishing AG, part of
Springer Nature 2018
J. S. Powers, *Value Driven Healthcare and Geriatric Medicine*,
https://doi.org/10.1007/978-3-319-77057-4_9

gibles are 65 years and older. [1]. Currently 10.4 million Medicare beneficiaries are also enrolled in the Medicaid program [2].

Of all the participants in Medicare and Medicaid, the dual-eligible population includes recipients who have the lowest incomes and highest chronic disease burden. Full duals as a group account for a disproportionate share of federal and state spending for Medicare and Medicaid. Full duals make up 13% of the combined population of Medicare enrollees and aged, blind, or disabled Medicaid enrollees (the categories of Medicaid participants who might also qualify for Medicare), but they account for 34% of the two programs' total spending on those enrollees [4]. Additionally for Medicare, duals represent 18% of the Medicare population but 32% of Medicare expenditures. Some 58% report functional ability deficits. Average per capita Medicare spending on dual-eligible beneficiaries was twice that for non-dual-eligible beneficiaries in 2013 ($19,785 compared to $9035) and 9% of duals live in institutional settings compared to 4% of non-dual-eligible Medicare beneficiaries [2]. The dual-eligible population has a high proportion of high-cost chronic conditions compared to other populations (Fig. 9.1). The dual-eligible population is by any measure a high-risk, high-need population.

In practice, Medicare functions as the primary insurance for acute medical care, including hospital, physician, and diagnostic services. Medicaid helps fill in many of the gaps for dual-eligible beneficiaries for care not covered by Medicare. Medicaid covers out-of-pocket costs associated with Medicare such as monthly premiums and cost-sharing amounts. However, state Medicaid programs are not required to pay the full share of the Medicare cost-sharing amount. The largest gap that is filled by Medicaid is the coverage of long-term care services and supports, such as non-skilled nursing home care. These services are not covered by Medicare. Depending on their income and assets, dual-eligible beneficiaries may qualify for full or partial Medicaid coverage.

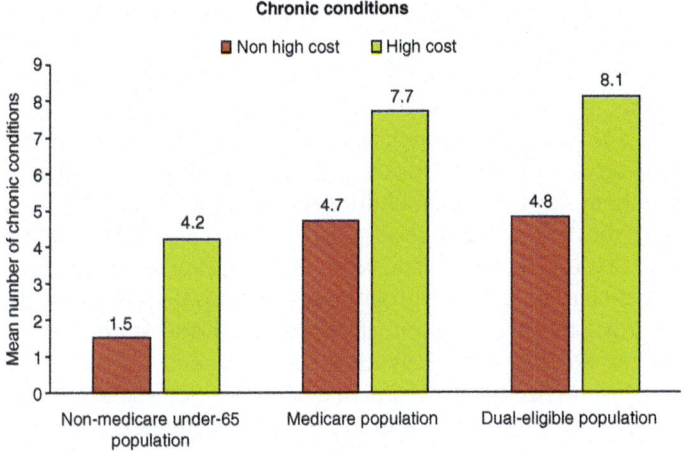

FIGURE 9.1 Mean number of chronic conditions among three groups of Massachusetts residents [3]

Medicaid is a state–federal partnership with policies driven at the state level through waivers and state plan amendments. To receive federal funding for Medicaid benefits, states must meet federal coverage standards, including covering designated populations like low-income older adults and providing a minimum set of covered benefits. The federal government provides matching funds to states for Medicaid funding. The matching rate ranges from 50% to about 75% across states depending on the state's economic circumstances, with wealthier states receiving a lower federal matching rate. Currently federal funding to states is guaranteed and fluctuates depending on program needs.

Beyond meeting the minimum federal Medicaid coverage standards for receiving federal matching funds, states can also opt to provide additional Medicaid benefits, such as dental services, or to expand coverage to additional populations, such as older adults who require long-term care services and supports but whose income is too high to otherwise qualify for Medicaid. States can also vary in how they administer their Medicaid benefits, including the setting of provider payment rates and requiring beneficiaries to join Medicaid managed care plans.

Cost sharing and benefits are shifted between the two programs, impacting access to care and quality of care. For example, a dual-eligible beneficiary who lives in a nursing home may rely on Medicare to cover all acute medical costs, such as inpatient stays and rehabilitative services, but rely on Medicaid to cover the long-term residential costs of living in the nursing home. It is difficult to achieve an optimal level of care for this beneficiary unless each program coordinates these services. To improve the organization of care, federal and state governments, working with their local partners, need to coordinate and incentivize the provision of evidence-based social support services in conjunction with the delivery of medical services.

In recent years, participation in managed care plans has been increasing for dual-eligible beneficiaries. For their Medicare benefits, dual-eligible beneficiaries can elect to enroll in managed care plans that are offered through the Medicare Advantage Program. In 2014, 2.8 million dual-eligible beneficiaries belonged to Medicare managed care plans [4]. Indeed, Congress authorized a unique set of plans called Dual-Eligible Special Needs Plans in 2003 that can exclusively enroll dual-eligible beneficiaries. These plans may improve care delivery by providing enhanced benefits, including care coordination services. In contrast to traditional Medicare, though, managed care plans can also implement narrow or restricted provider networks and employ practices like prior authorization, which may limit their popularity with dual-eligible beneficiaries.

For the provision of Medicaid benefits, states can require their dual-eligible beneficiaries to enroll in managed care plans that administer Medicaid benefits, including long-term care services and supports. As of 2014, 17 states required that dual-eligible beneficiaries enroll in Medicaid managed care plans [4]. An additional 26 states gave dual-eligible beneficiaries the option of enrolling in a Medicaid managed care plan. As of 2013 there were some 272 Medicaid managed care organizations operating nationally [5].

Managed care plans have been viewed as a pathway for providing more integrated care delivery and for aligning financial incentives across Medicare and Medicaid to achieve better care coordination and quality of care. One such model is a voluntary integration approach where dual-eligible beneficiaries choose to enroll in a Medicaid managed care plan and a Medicare managed care plan operated by the same insurer. Although the beneficiary is enrolled in two separate plans, the insurer has a financial incentive to efficiently coordinate Medicaid and Medicare benefits. This minimizes regulatory duplication and differences between Medicare and Medicaid while streamlining processes such as enrollment and data reporting. A second approach, which is being tested by the federal government and select states, involves creating managed care plans that contract with Medicare and a state Medicaid program to provide Medicare and Medicaid benefits through a unified plan. These plans must achieve certain quality standards. Because these plans are paid on a capitated basis, they can financially benefit from any savings in providing improved quality and reduced cost for Medicare/Medicaid recipients [6].

Medicaid allows waivers for states to implement demonstration programs demonstrating value-based purchasing to improve service outcomes for duals. Many adults in the dual population have multiple illnesses that require intensive care coordination. Access to behavioral health remains limited in many communities however and functional limitations combined with limited transportation interfere with access producing challenges to obtaining quality care for many duals.

Low reimbursement rates may make it difficult to attract managed care organizations to participate in capitated dual-eligible demonstrations. A Federal Coordinated Healthcare Office (FCHCO) has been developed to assist duals in obtaining access to entitled services, to simplify enrollment processes for long-term care and social support services, and to encourage improved provider performance under the Medicare and Medicaid programs.

Provision of care to the dual-eligible population depends heavily on the structure of healthcare financing, determinations of eligibility, and both federal and state funding. Thus these programs are at risk depending on political considerations. Changes in access and eligibility and any resultant disparity among states could profoundly affect quality metrics and consequently the health of the dual-eligible population. Medicaid consumes a growing share of state budgets as the number of enrollees grows. As much as 70% of program resources are devoted to individuals with disabilities living in institutional settings. An interactive site displaying data for each state Medicaid program in summary fashion is available at the Kaiser Family Foundation website [7].

The cost of home services is low for individuals requiring basic care but as added services are imported into the home the cost could easily exceed the cost of nursing home care. Some states use a needs assessment tied to functional abilities and may restrict home- and community-based services, possibly forcing some individuals into long-term care facilities. For example, Tennessee's Medicaid program requires functional disability equivalent to nursing home admission criteria, but limits care at home to less than the cost of nursing home care [8].

Medicaid has been an open-ended entitlement program extremely popular with beneficiaries and the general public [9]. Subject to program rules, states can receive matching funds on their Medicaid spending without limit. Changes in Medicaid funding including Medicaid block grants, whether capitated or fixed, could give states more flexibility, but also put them at risk for covering increasing healthcare costs. States could respond and severely limit Medicaid services. Less funding could be available for mental health services and home and community-based care. Block grants could also lock in historical differences between states increasing disparities and reducing reimbursement to providers including physicians, hospitals, and long-term care facilities, thus further reducing access for vulnerable populations.

There are calls to reform Medicaid to help improve enrollment and coordination [10] and to provide outcome-based core program metrics [11]. Outcome metrics could help guide Medicaid program quality and balance resource allocation decisions.

References

1. Congressional Budget Office. Dual-Eligible Beneficiaries of Medicare and Medicaid: Characteristics, Health Care Spending, and Evolving Policies. https://www.cbo.gov/sites/default/files/113th-congress-2013-2014/reports/44308dualeligibles2.pdf. Accessed 17 Nov 2017.
2. Medicare Payment Advisory Commission. Data book: Beneficiaries dually eligible for Medicare and Medicaid — June 2017 MedPAC | MACPAC. http://www.medpac.gov/docs/default-source/data-book/jun17_databookentirereport_sec.pdf?sfvrsn=0. Accessed 17 Nov 2017.
3. National Academy of Medicine. Effective care for high need patients: opportunities for improving outcomes, value, and health. Ch 2. Key characteristics of high need patients. https://nam.edu/initiatives/clinician-resilience-and-well-being/effective-care-for-high-need-patients/. Accessed 17 Nov 2017.
4. Centers for Medicare and Medicaid Services. CMS Program Statistics, 2014 Medicare enrollment section https://www.cms.gov/Research-Statistics-Data-and-Systems/Statistics-Trends-and-Reports/CMSProgramStatistics/2014/2014_Enrollment.html. Accessed 17 Nov 2017.
5. Ndumeie CD, Schpero WL, Schlesinger MJ, Trivedi AN. Association between health plan exit from Medicaid managed care and quality of care, 2006–2014. JAMA. 2017;317:524–2531.
6. Warshaw G, DeGolia PA. Medicare and medicaid coordination: special case of the dual eligible beneficiaries. In: Powers JS, editor. Healthcare changes and the affordable care act. Switzerland: Springer International Publishing; 2015. p. 117–32.
7. Henry J Kaiser Family Foundation, Medicaid state fact sheets http://kff.org/interactive/medicaid-state-fact-sheets/. Accessed 17 Nov 2017.

8. TennCare Choices program eligibility sheet. https://www.tn.gov/tenncare/article/to-qualify-for-choices. Accessed 17 Nov 2017.
9. Inglehart JK, Sommers BD. Medicaid at 50: from welfare program to nations largest health insurer. N Engl J Med. 2015;372:2152–9.
10. Branch E, Bella M. What is the focus of the integrated care initiatives aimed at Medicare-Medicaid beneficiaries? J Amer Soc Aging. 2013;37:6–12.
11. Slavitt A, Wilensky G. JAMA forum: reforming Medicaid. JAMA. 2017;318:601–2.

Chapter 10
Through the Looking Glass: Visions of the Future of Health Care

Abstract The value-based transformation of the US health-care system is here to stay. Expectations regarding quality, transparency, standardization, and cost control will be permanent fixtures. How the healthcare system responds to change remains to be seen. The potential to analyze large amounts of health-related data promises to improve patient care by informing care decisions and evaluating treatment effectiveness. Implementation of new practices has the potential to improve the standards of care. Health care can become a new partnership with patients as key stakeholders engaged in personal responsibility for their own health.

Scope of the Problem

Healthcare transformation has dramatically changed the healthcare landscape. These include three major considerations: (1) access, (2) quality, and (3) cost control.

Access issues are politically highly charged as they relate to government influence regarding healthcare disparities, an individual mandate for health insurance coverage, uniform health benefits, and exclusion of preexisting conditions in adjusting premiums. Most medical organizations and the majority of the public favor public support for healthcare coverage [1]. The Congressional Budget Office estimates that

© Springer International Publishing AG, part of   137
Springer Nature 2018
J. S. Powers, *Value Driven Healthcare and Geriatric Medicine*,
https://doi.org/10.1007/978-3-319-77057-4_10

the elimination of the individual mandate for health insurance, which takes effect in 2019, will increase the pool of uninsured individuals by 13 million, and increase premiums by 10% for all, as younger healthy individuals are no longer required to purchase insurance [2]. Many elderly individuals could have much higher premiums, as the marketplace dictates. Medicaid, which covers 20% of the population, could be block-granted to the states, shifting more costs to individual states. Millions of individuals may forgo health insurance if it is unaffordable, and the array of services covered by Medicaid could be dramatically reduced by individual states.

Regarding provision of quality care, this element has broad support and is likely to be a permanent fixture of health care. Quality outcomes are the core of value-based purchasing as reflected in the quality reporting metrics for hospitals and physicians, the new transparent Physician Compare site which the public can access, and the payment incentives for systems and physicians. The Medicare Access and Children's Health Insurance Program Reauthorization Act (MACRA) has replaced the Medicare Sustainable Growth Rate (SGR) formula for physician payment, and physicians can retain bonuses for achieving quality performance, reflected in an increase in the Medicare reimbursement rate (up to 4%). Clinicians are increasingly encouraged to participate in new models of care and advanced alternative payment models (APMs) and realize a 5% increase in Part B Medicare reimbursement. Publicly reported quality metrics may also be a condition for participation in health plans, maintenance of licensure, liability coverage, or inclusion in group practices. Quality reporting could be a very powerful lever for behavior change among providers, healthcare organizations, and consumers, reducing regional variation in Medicare spending, and forcing individual physicians to adhere to consensus guidelines and standards of care.

There is also very broad support regarding cost control. While healthcare inflation has been moderated since 2010, there is evidence that healthcare costs are beginning to rise again. The value transformation of health care represents a paradigm shift. Early findings suggest that value-based purchasing has helped to moderate healthcare costs, but it only represents a small portion of the entire healthcare economy at this time. Health spending is projected to grow 1.2 percentage points faster than the gross domestic project (GDP) per year over 2016–2025; as a result, the health share of GDP is expected to rise from 17.8% in 2015 to 19.9% by 2025 [2]. If value-based transformation cannot control medical inflation and keep the rate of increase of healthcare expenditures to less than the GDP, there is strong support for further price cutting for hospitals, pharmaceuticals, and physicians [3]. In order to accelerate the adoption of advanced APMs, the Medicare Payment Advisory Commission (MedPAC) could also create an alternative Voluntary Value Program to encourage clinicians to form voluntary groups and reward them for population-based outcomes from a pool of fee schedule dollars withheld from Medicare providers. Federal reductions in Medicare funding could further affect prices paid to providers as well as suppliers.

It is also possible that individuals are taking more responsibility for their health, as insurance premiums have increased for all. Part of this is due to shifting of cost to consumers by insurance companies who now have their profits limited—tied to an 85% loss ratio (limit of 15% overhead and profit) for larger firms. The loss ratio is 80% for smaller insurers. Increased healthcare benefits (minimum mandatory benefits) have also contributed to increased insurance costs. Employers providing health insurance to workers are also shifting some of this cost to consumers. Consumers will want to reduce their premiums, therefore popularizing higher deductible plans. The increased visibility of healthcare costs now shared directly with the consumer may be contributing to increased personal responsibility for health and health behaviors, and this may help moderate future healthcare costs.

Challenges Ahead

Trainees aspiring to specialty-oriented careers are still functioning in a fee-for-service (FFS) model and mindset. But the planned demise of FFS is real and medical societies and individual practitioners will have difficulty adopting new models and changing from traditional operating procedures. Medical societies and educators need to help. The focus on quality and cost control is likely to be permanent features of the healthcare landscape. FFS is being phased out as practitioners are encouraged to join advanced APMs.

There is an immediate need for the healthcare system to respond and change. Starting in 2018 CMS will calculate cost measures using claims data at the level of the provider or group and evaluations will occur on measures relevant to these practices. Provider choices of quality measures will have to be strategic and specialty appropriate. Global healthcare system budgeting and value-based purchasing and stimulation of new healthcare models will be emphasized. Cost-avoidance strategies are becoming the new cost centers.

Adapting to a new healthcare system will involve individual and health system providers, educators, and increased patient-centered personal health decisions and responsibility. Geriatrics and care of older adults will have a profound effect on the shaping of the healthcare system of the future [4]. We need to change the conversation to promote optimal aging and change the culture of how we as a society regard aging and what it means to grow older. We need to create an inclusive, intergenerational society which accepts continuing to live and age in a positive light. There is no controversy about the fact that society is indeed aging and our healthcare system must respond appropriately [5]. New models of care including team-based health care, global budgeting, and bundling of services are expected to increase in importance and acceptance. These changes will dramatically influence medical education as we prepare new practitioners for a new healthcare environment. Oversight and public accountability of healthcare training are also expected to increase as society needs physicians and health systems which are able to meet consumer needs in a new value-based environment.

Response to Change

The complexity of the issues posed by changes in health care and medicine that our society needs to address is so enormous that no sector can devise solutions on its own. Some have argued that the changes required are so profound that a single-payer health system may be required to facilitate this process. A single-payer system is consistent with value-based purchasing and is one means to achieve universal healthcare coverage. A review of single-payer models for the United States shows many heterogeneous proposals to achieve this end, utilizing both public and private resources [6].

Professional providers and health systems interact with the health insurance industry providing managed care products in a preferred provider relationship. This could cause providers to act in unacceptable ways, creating moral hazards. While patient-centered care causes the physician to provide services in consideration of patient needs, managed care on the other hand may cause providers to deny services on the basis of cost and best interest of the third-party payer or the provider. Currently there is little oversight and the current legal system is inadequate when applied to the relationship between providers, third-party payers, and consumers. We need to act with care when designing utilization review programs and giving financial incentives to providers to ensure that choices made are in the best interest of the patient.

Big data holds the potential to analyze large amounts of health-related information to apply to patient care with the promise for improving care by better informing care decisions, increasing treatment safety, and more accurately evaluating treatment effectiveness. Big data analytics has historically been less utilized in health care compared to other industries due to confidentiality concerns, but this is changing. While appropriate statistical methods will be needed to control for potential bias in interpreting data sets collected for purposes other than the specific clinical and process questions posed, the benefit of big data to enhance the patient-centered approach to care is enormous. Big data can identify valuable pathways to identify new therapies and approaches to help patients achieve better outcomes. It can provide data to personalize interventions, monitor for complications, communicate with patients, and information resources for precision medicine. Precision medicine aims to link large data sets related to prognosis, treatments, risk, and monitoring of progress for individual patients to help clinicians personalize care. Big data analytics can improve population management and follow health trends, as well as evaluate models of care. Harnessing these capabilities can advance continuous clinical learning and research which draws on real-world evidence. To maximize this potential, we must partner with patients and families to support the sharing of health information.

Harmonization of performance and quality measures among healthcare professionals, healthcare organizations, health plans, and CMS through public reporting can speed the implementation of new practices and create clear expectations of practice behavior, improving standards of care. Standards of care can be an important lever for rapid integration of evidence and new clinical standards into practice. This provides a great opportunity for clinical leadership. We need committed physician leaders who are able to coach colleagues, evaluate outcome data, and guide practice changes [7].

The electronic health record (EHR), intended for improved patient care, is often criticized as having unintended

TABLE 10.1 Novel metrics for an improved EHR [8]

- Work after work—this measures EHR logons and tasks during evenings, weekends, and vacations

- Click counts—this counts the number of clicks needed to accomplish common workflow tasks and is a key measure of usability

- Teamwork-related measures—tracking a ratio of staff entered to the physician-entered EHR tasks to identify how well tasks are distributed to the appropriate team members

- Being present—this metric tracks the proportion of time spent with the patient versus EHR documentation during a visit

- Fair pay—these metrics track generally uncompensated work such as managing messages and e-mails, providing medication refills, as well as managing patient-generated health data to highlight EHR-related administrative work that creates value for patient care

- Regulatory balance—these measures relate to pay for performance-related EHR activities or billing-related documentation

consequences impairing practice efficiency. In order to provide adequate support and usable EHR tools, novel metrics have been proposed to capture the facilitators of and impediments to patient care [8]. These proposed new metrics are displayed in Table 10.1.

Improving usability of EHR tasks which complete for physician attention during the visit is important for professional satisfaction as well as for improved patient care. Measurement of EHR metrics is important to the provider to help drive patient-centered improvements and future modifications of the EHR.

The shift in healthcare culture toward value-based care requires thinking outside of the FFS box. Using an Agency for Healthcare Research and Quality (AHRQ) algorithm to identify potentially preventable hospitalizations and ED visits for 2012 Medicare data, some 4.8% of Medicare spending was found to be potentially preventable. Of this, 73.8% was incurred by high-cost patients. Despite making up only 4% of the Medicare population, high-cost, frail elderly patients accounted for 43.9% of potentially preventable spending [9]. As organizations take on financial risk for patients, it is important to provide high-value care for these high-need, high-cost older adults. It is important to better understand this diverse population, identify evidence-based programs that offer higher quality, integrated care at lower cost, and intensify both incentives and support for clinicians to adopt and continue to improve higher value methods of managing high-need high-cost populations [10, 11].

Educators for future healthcare professionals have a huge task ahead to prepare them for effective practice models in a transformed value-based healthcare system. Future clinicians need to be able to respond professionally to new care models and management of health-related data. Virtual care, new team-based models of care, and value-based purchasing will produce new healthcare professional roles and behavior [12]. We need to revitalize primary care and enhance appreciation for the critical and complex role it plays. We must implement initiatives for clinicians to build patient-centered skill sets for engagement, shared decision-making, and better definitions of value reflecting the patient perspective while determining appropriate measures for evaluation of those skills. There needs to be greater oversight of healthcare training focused on societal needs.

It is critical to prepare the workforce to deliver team-based, comprehensive health care. We need to develop training and certification opportunities focusing on the treatment and social support needs of high-need patients, including care coordination. Credentialing programs for nontraditional healthcare workers such as community health workers and peer support providers should also be developed [13].

Facility with quality improvement is critical to future practitioners as they set standards for practice. The ability to integrate data into practice and to continue to refresh the clinical approach is a highly desirable skill. Future practitioners need tools to speed the introduction and evaluation of innovations into practice.

Patients must be informed regarding healthcare advances including the appropriate use, value, potential harms, and potential financial obligations. We need to equip patients and families as partners and stakeholders. They need to be heard, understood, and involved in their care. Personal health choices and responsibility are enhanced with value-based healthcare transformation, risk sharing, and scope of personal responsibility for health care.

Patient decision aides include printed booklets, videos, and Web-based tools created for patients that provide evidence-based information on the options available for a specific health condition including benefits and harms for each option. They allow patients to consider what is important and permit them to establish their preferred screening or treatment options. Patient decision aides help provide shared decision-making whereby clinicians and patients work together to understand the patient's situation and better determine how best to address it. Systematic reviews of shared decision-making found that patient decision aides are associated with improved decision quality and decision-making processes without worse patient or healthcare outcomes. However, little is known about the effect of patient decision aides on patient competence with decision-making, cost, resource use, or adherence to selected options [14, 15]. Additional study is needed to know the extent to which these tools improve the patient's sense of intellectual, emotional, and practical involvement in their own care, and encourage new ways to promote patient involvement in making important healthcare decisions. We also need to improve the quality of communication between healthcare professionals and patients living with serious illness through a broad range of research covering communication skills, tools, patient education, and models of care [16]. New EHR products can provide printed patient educational materials pertinent to the patients' encounter as part of the visit summary. Patient EHR portals may enhance communication and patient engagement in their own care.

More patient engagement, home monitoring of health status, and increased participation in one's own care could help maintain population health status. Appropriate medical utilization could decrease in the presence of barriers such as limited access, financial constraints, and provider availability.

Patients must be engaged and provided opportunity to give input for patient-centered products, services, and models of care. Quality measures should include measures that truly capture what patients care about. While consensus among experts, advocacy groups, payers, and consumers regarding what constitutes high-value measures and how best to measure them may be difficult to achieve, a small number of high-value measures would help force hospitals and providers to become flexible and truly patient centered by meeting the varying needs and values of patients [17].

Patients also need to be engaged so that outcomes measure what matters most. Capturing overall caregiver and patient experience and perceived quality of care is of great importance for every patient and every care setting. The joint American Academy of Hospice and Palliative Medicine and the Hospice and Palliative Nurses Association's Measuring What Matters (MWM) initiative identified a number of quality indicators for hospice and palliative care practice, including treatment preferences, care consistent with documented care preferences, global measure of patient experience, and respect for cultural aspects of care [18]. Measuring what matters most is critical to understanding quality by measuring what is important to patients, families, and also providers. We greatly need identification, implementation, and tracking of metrics that can be used to inform quality of processes, which are validated in different populations and practice settings, in order to strengthen the linkages between these process measures and patient and caregiver outcomes [19].

We need to know what patients are willing to contribute to their health in the forms of copayments and deductibles, traditionally considered to be barriers to healthcare access. A recent study of cost sharing and utilization of home care services among Medicare advantage enrollees found no evidence that imposing copayments reduces the use of home health services among older adults. More intensive use of home health services was associated with increased rates of disenrollment from Medicare advantage plans, although the duration of home care was similar among traditional to care and Medicare advantage enrollees [20].

Electronic health data are expanding to now include patient-reported outcomes, patient-generated health data, and social determinants of health. Enabling access to personal health data may benefit patients as well as healthcare professionals and increase patient engagement, data accuracy, and perhaps health outcomes. Enhancements to the EHR to improve interoperability will include (1) standardized common data elements enabling the sharing and emerging of health data from multiple sources, (2) patient encounter data receipts automatically pushed to the patient's digital health record, and (3) a data use agreement (DUA) between patients and healthcare organizations enabling individuals to control their longitudinal electronic health record [21].

Looking to the Future

We should accept the advent of value-based healthcare transformation and appropriately adapt and accommodate relevant business, education, and practice models. The promise of an improved healthcare experience, quality of care, and cost control is real. Health care then becomes a new partnership with patients as key stakeholders.

References

1. Kaiser Family Foundation poll: Future of the Affordable Care Act. http://kff.org/health-reform/report/kaiser-health-tracking-poll-late-april-2017-the-future-of-the-aca-and-health-care-the-budget/. Accessed 17 Nov 2017.
2. Congressional Budget Office. Repealing the individual health insurance mandate: an updated estimate, November 8, 2017. https://www.cbo.gov/publication/53300. Accessed 21 Dec 2017.

3. Cutler DM. Rising costs mean more rough times ahead. JAMA. 2107;318:508–9.
4. Tinetti M. Mainstream or extinction: can defining who we are save geriatrics? J Am Geriatr Soc. 2016;64:1400–4.
5. Jenkins JA. Disrupt Aging. A bold new path to living your best life at every age. New York: Public Affairs Publishers; 2016.
6. Liu J, Brook RH. What is single-payer healthcare. A review of the definitions and proposals in the US. J Gen Int Med. 2017;32:822–31.
7. Rosenblatt M, Austin CP, Boutin M, et al. Innovation in development, regulatory review, and use of clinical advances: a vital direction for health and health care. Washington, DC: National Academy of Medicine; 2016.
8. DiAngi YT, Lee TC, Sinsky CA, Bohman BD, Sharp CD. Novel metrics for improving professional fulfillment. Ann Intern Med. 2017;167:740–1.
9. Figueroa JF, Joynt Maddox KE, Beaulieu N, Wild RC, Jha AK. Concentration of potentially preventable spending among high-cost of Medicare subpopulations. Ann Intern Med. 2017;167:706–13.
10. Leff B, Milstein A. Possibilities beyond analysis of a fee-for-service database and clinician mindset. Ann Intern Med. 2017;167:746–7.
11. Blumenthal D, Chernof B, Fulmer T, Lumpkin J, Selberg J. Caring for high-need, high-cost patients–an urgent priority. N Engl J Med. 2016;375:909–11.
12. Duval JF, Opas LM, Nasca TJ, et al. Envisioning the sponsoring institution of the future: report of the SI2025 task force. J Grad Med Ed. 2017;9(6 suppl 1):11–57.
13. Thomas-Henkel C, Hamblin A, Hendricks T. Opportunities to improve models of care for people with complex needs. Princeton, NJ: Robert Wood Johnson Foundation & Center for Health Care Strategies; 2015.
14. Stacey D, Legare F, Lewis K, et al. Decision aides for people facing health treatment or screening decisions. Cochrane Database Syst Rev. 2017;4:CD0001431.
15. Shay LA, Lafata JE. What is the evidence? A systematic review of shared decision making and patient outcomes. Med Decision Making. 2015;35:114–31.
16. Tulsky JA, Beach MC, Butow PH, et al. A research agenda for communication between healthcare professionals and patients living with serious illness. JAMA Intern Med. 2017;117:1361–6.

17. Jha AK. Payment power to the patients. JAMA. 2017;318:18–9.
18. Dy SM, Kiley KB, Ast K, et al. Measuring what matters: top-ranked quality indicators for hospice and palliative care from the American Academy of Hospice and Palliative Medicine and Hospice and Palliative Nurses Association. JPSM. 2015;49:773–81.
19. Unroe KT, Ast K, Chuang E, Schulman-Green D, Gramling R, AAHPM Research Committee Writing Group. The implementation of measuring what matters in research and practice: series commentary. JPSM. 2017;54:772–5.
20. Li Q, Keohane LM, Lee Y, Trivedi AN. Association of cost sharing with use of home health services among Medicare advantage enrollees. JAMA Intern Med. 2017;177:1012–8.
21. Mikk KA, Sleeper HA, Topol EJ. The pathway to patient data ownership and better health. JAMA. 2017;318:1433–4.

Index

The manufacturer's authorised representative in the EU is Springer
Nature Customer Service Centre GmbH, Europaplatz 3, 69115 Heidelberg,
Germany. If you have any concerns regarding our products, please
contact ProductSafety@springernature.com

Printed and bound by CPI Group (UK) Ltd, Croydon, CR0 4YY
27/04/2026
02097580-0001